AYURVEDIC WISDOM:
BALANCING BODY, MIND, AND SPIRIT

© Copyright 2024 by Serenity Sagewood - All rights reserved.

It is not legal to reproduce, duplicate, or transmit any part of this document in either electronic means or printed format. Recording of this publication is strictly prohibited.

Preface

After the release of "Beyond Conventional: The Complete Guide to Alternative and Holistic Health," I was overwhelmed by the positive feedback and the numerous requests from readers who wished to delve deeper into specific aspects of holistic practices. The desire for more detailed guidance and the enthusiasm for exploring ancient wisdom in our modern world inspired me to embark on this new journey.

This book, "Ayurvedic Wisdom: Balancing Body, Mind, and Spirit," is the first in a series aimed at providing a comprehensive exploration of various holistic methods. Ayurveda, with its rich history and profound understanding of the human body and mind, felt like the perfect starting point. It offers timeless insights and practical tools that can be seamlessly integrated into our daily lives, promoting balance, health, and well-being.

In this book, I have strived to present the principles of Ayurveda in an accessible and practical manner. Whether you are new to Ayurveda or seeking to deepen your knowledge, this guide will serve as a valuable resource on your journey to holistic health.

I am excited to share this deeper dive into Ayurvedic practices with you, and I hope it enriches your life as much as it has mine.

With gratitude,

Serenity Sagewood

Chapter 1:
Introduction to Ayurveda

Ayurveda, often referred to as the "Science of Life," is one of the world's oldest systems of natural medicine, rooted in the ancient Indian subcontinent. It is more than just a medical system; Ayurveda is a holistic approach to health and wellness that encompasses the balance of the body, mind, and spirit. This chapter will introduce you to the fundamental aspects of Ayurveda, exploring its origins, core principles, and relevance in today's fast-paced world. As we delve into this ancient wisdom, you'll begin to see how Ayurveda can serve as a guiding light on your journey to holistic well-being.

The Origins of Ayurveda

Historical Background

The origins of Ayurveda can be traced back over 5,000 years to the ancient Indian civilization. It is said to have been passed down orally from the gods to sages and then to human physicians. The earliest references to Ayurvedic principles can be found in the Vedas, the ancient Hindu scriptures. Specifically, the Atharva Veda contains hymns and prayers that detail medicinal practices and the use of herbs, which laid the groundwork for what would eventually become Ayurveda.

The development of Ayurveda was not just a matter of accumulating knowledge but involved a deep understanding of the human body, mind, and spirit. The sages who developed Ayurveda were keen observers of nature and the human condition, and they used this knowledge to create a system of healing that is both comprehensive and adaptable.

During the Vedic period, Ayurveda was integrated into the daily lives of people, influencing everything from diet and lifestyle to spiritual practices. The sages recognized that health is not merely the absence of disease but a state of complete physical, mental, and spiritual well-being. This holistic approach is what sets Ayurveda apart from many other medical systems.

As Ayurveda evolved, it became an integral part of Indian culture and society. It was practiced not only by healers and physicians but also by ordinary people who followed Ayurvedic principles to maintain their health and prevent disease. This widespread practice helped to preserve and transmit Ayurvedic knowledge through generations, ensuring its survival even in the face of challenges such as invasions and colonization.

Foundational Texts and Scholars

The most significant contributions to Ayurveda come from two ancient texts: the Charaka Samhita and the Sushruta Samhita. These texts, composed between 1000 BCE and 500 CE, are considered the primary sources of Ayurvedic knowledge.

The Charaka Samhita, attributed to the sage Charaka, is a comprehensive treatise on internal medicine. It outlines various aspects of diagnosis, treatment, and the holistic approach to health, emphasizing the importance of diet, lifestyle, and mental well-being in maintaining health. Charaka's teachings stress the importance of understanding the root cause of disease rather than just treating symptoms. He also emphasized the role of the physician's intuition and insight in the healing process, a concept that resonates with modern ideas of personalized medicine.

The Sushruta Samhita, attributed to the sage Sushruta, focuses on surgery and the treatment of injuries. It is one of the earliest works to detail surgical procedures, including the use of anesthesia, sutures, and surgical instruments. Sushruta is often referred to as the "father of surgery" for his contributions to this field. His work highlights the advanced understanding of anatomy and surgical techniques that existed in ancient India. The text includes descriptions of various surgical instruments, procedures for treating fractures and wounds, and even methods for reconstructive surgery, such as rhinoplasty.

Another important text is the Ashtanga Hridaya, a concise compilation of Ayurvedic principles and practices by the sage

Vagbhata. This text is widely regarded for its clarity and practical approach, making it a popular reference for both practitioners and students of Ayurveda. Vagbhata's work is known for its emphasis on the importance of maintaining balance in all aspects of life, from diet and exercise to mental and emotional health.

These foundational texts were further expanded upon by other scholars over the centuries, leading to a rich tradition of Ayurvedic knowledge that has been preserved and passed down through generations. The continuity of Ayurvedic practice is a testament to its effectiveness and adaptability. Despite the passage of time, the core principles of Ayurveda remain as relevant today as they were thousands of years ago.

Principles of Ayurvedic Philosophy

Understanding the Five Elements

At the core of Ayurvedic philosophy lies the concept of the five elements, or Panchamahabhutas. These elements—Earth (Prithvi), Water (Jala), Fire (Agni), Air (Vayu), and Ether (Akasha)—are considered the building blocks of the universe. According to Ayurveda, everything in the physical world, including the human body, is composed of these five elements in varying proportions.

Each element represents different qualities and functions. For example, Earth symbolizes stability and structure, while Fire represents transformation and metabolism. Water is associated with fluidity and cohesion, Air with movement and dynamism, and Ether with space and potential. Understanding the interplay of these elements within our bodies and the environment is key to maintaining balance and health.

The concept of the five elements is not just theoretical; it has practical applications in understanding the human body and its functions. For instance, the Earth element is associated with the bones and muscles, providing structure and support. The Water element is linked to bodily fluids, such as blood and lymph, which nourish and cleanse the body. The Fire element governs digestion and metabolism, transforming food into energy. The Air element controls the respiratory and circulatory systems, enabling movement and communication within the body. Finally, the Ether element is connected to the spaces within the body, such as the cavities of the lungs and the digestive tract, allowing for the transmission of energy and information.

The Concept of Doshas

Building on the concept of the five elements, Ayurveda introduces the idea of doshas, which are the fundamental energies governing physiological activity within the body. There are three primary doshas: Vata, Pitta, and Kapha, each corresponding to a combination of two elements.

- **Vata (Air and Ether):** Vata is responsible for movement, including the circulation of blood, the flow of breath, and the transmission of nerve impulses. It governs creativity and flexibility but can lead to anxiety and restlessness when out of balance. Individuals with a dominant Vata dosha are often quick thinkers, lively, and energetic, but they may also be prone to dryness, coldness, and irregularity in their bodily functions.

- **Pitta (Fire and Water):** Pitta governs transformation, including digestion, metabolism, and body temperature. It is associated with intelligence and courage, but an imbalance can result in anger, irritation, and inflammation. Pitta individuals tend to be driven, focused, and competitive, with strong digestion and a warm body temperature. However, excess Pitta can lead to issues such as acidity, inflammation, and irritability.

- **Kapha (Earth and Water):** Kapha provides structure and stability, governing the body's tissues, immunity, and fluid balance. It is linked to calmness and loyalty but can lead to lethargy and attachment when imbalanced. People with a dominant Kapha dosha are often steady, nurturing, and resilient, with a tendency to accumulate weight and retain water. When out of balance, Kapha can cause sluggishness, congestion, and a lack of motivation.

Each person is born with a unique combination of these doshas, known as their Prakriti, which determines their physical and mental characteristics. This inherent constitution influences everything from body type and personality to dietary preferences and susceptibility to certain illnesses. Understanding your dominant dosha can help you make lifestyle choices that support your health and well-being.

In Ayurveda, the goal is to maintain a balance among the doshas. Imbalances can occur due to various factors, such as improper diet, stress, seasonal changes, or environmental influences. When the doshas are out of balance, it can lead to physical and mental discomfort, and eventually, disease. By recognizing the signs of dosha imbalance, you can take steps to restore harmony through diet, lifestyle modifications, and Ayurvedic treatments.

Relevance of Ayurveda Today

Modern Applications

Despite its ancient origins, Ayurveda remains highly relevant in today's world. As modern society faces an increasing number of health challenges, including chronic stress, lifestyle-related diseases, and a disconnect from nature, Ayurveda offers practical solutions that are both timeless and adaptable.

One of the key strengths of Ayurveda is its focus on prevention. By promoting balance and harmony in all aspects of life, Ayurveda helps individuals avoid illness before it manifests. This proactive approach contrasts with the reactive nature of many modern medical systems, which often focus on treating symptoms rather than addressing underlying causes.

Ayurveda's emphasis on holistic health means that it considers not just the physical body but also the mind and spirit. In a world where mental health issues are on the rise, Ayurveda's integrated approach offers valuable insights into maintaining emotional and psychological well-being. Practices such as meditation, yoga, and mindful breathing, which are integral to Ayurveda, have gained widespread recognition for their effectiveness in reducing stress and enhancing mental clarity.

Ayurveda also emphasizes the importance of individualized care. Recognizing that each person is unique, it provides tailored recommendations for diet, exercise, and lifestyle based on an individual's dosha constitution. This personalized approach ensures that health practices are aligned with one's natural tendencies, leading to more sustainable results.

In recent years, there has been a growing interest in natural and holistic health practices, driven by concerns over the side effects of conventional medicine and the desire for more sustainable and eco-friendly solutions. Ayurveda, with its focus on natural remedies, dietary adjustments, and lifestyle changes, aligns well with these trends. Many people are turning to Ayurvedic practices to manage chronic conditions, enhance their quality of life, and achieve a greater sense of balance and well-being.

Integrating Ayurveda into Daily Life

Integrating Ayurvedic principles into your daily life doesn't require a complete overhaul of your current lifestyle. Instead, it involves making small, mindful changes that promote balance and well-being. This could be as simple as adjusting your diet to include more foods that pacify your dominant dosha, incorporating daily routines (Dinacharya) that align with natural rhythms, or using herbal remedies to support your health.

Ayurveda encourages living in harmony with nature, which includes aligning your activities with the cycles of the day and seasons. For example, waking up with the sunrise, eating your largest meal at midday when digestion is strongest, and winding down in the evening can all help you maintain balance. These practices are not just about physical health; they also support mental and emotional well-being by reducing stress and promoting a sense of calm and stability.

In addition to daily routines, Ayurveda offers guidance on seasonal adjustments. The changing seasons can have a significant impact on your dosha balance, and Ayurveda provides strategies for adapting your diet, lifestyle, and activities to stay in harmony with the environment. For example, during the dry and cold Vata season, you might focus on warming, nourishing foods and activities that promote grounding and relaxation. In the hot and intense Pitta season, you could incorporate cooling practices and foods to maintain balance.

Incorporating Ayurvedic practices into your life is a journey, not a destination. As you begin to explore this ancient wisdom, you'll discover new ways to enhance your well-being, build resilience against stress, and cultivate a deeper connection with yourself and the world around you. The beauty of Ayurveda lies in its adaptability and the way it empowers you to take charge of your health. Whether you're looking to address specific health issues or simply seeking a more balanced and fulfilling life, Ayurveda offers a wealth of knowledge and tools to support your journey.

In this chapter, we've explored the origins of Ayurveda, the foundational principles that underlie this ancient system, and its relevance in the modern world. We have seen how Ayurveda's holistic approach to health, with its emphasis on balance, prevention, and individualized care, continues to offer valuable insights and practices for maintaining well-being in today's fast-paced and often stressful environment.

As we move forward, we will dive deeper into the specific aspects of Ayurveda, starting with an in-depth exploration of the doshas in the next chapter. Understanding your unique dosha constitution is the first step in tailoring Ayurvedic practices to suit your individual needs and achieving greater balance in your life. By gaining a deeper understanding of the doshas, you'll be better equipped to make informed choices that support your health and well-being on all levels—body, mind, and spirit.

Chapter 2: Understanding the Doshas

In Ayurveda, understanding the doshas is central to achieving and maintaining health. The doshas—Vata, Pitta, and Kapha—are the fundamental energies that govern all physiological and psychological processes in the human body. They are derived from the five elements and manifest in unique combinations within each individual, creating a personal constitution, or Prakriti, that influences everything from body type to temperament. This chapter will explore the characteristics of each dosha, the implications of dosha imbalances, and how to determine your own dosha. By understanding the doshas, you can tailor Ayurvedic practices to your specific needs, promoting harmony and well-being in your life.

The Three Doshas Explained

Vata: The Energy of Movement

Vata is the dosha associated with the elements of Air and Ether, making it the force responsible for all movement in the body and mind. It governs essential functions such as circulation, respiration, nerve impulses, and the flow of thoughts. Vata is light, dry, cold, and mobile, and these qualities are reflected in individuals who have a dominant Vata constitution.

People with a Vata-dominant Prakriti are often characterized by a lean and slender build, with dry skin and hair. They tend to be creative, energetic, and quick-witted, but can also be prone to anxiety, restlessness, and insomnia when out of balance. Vata types are often highly active, both mentally and physically, but they may struggle with staying grounded and maintaining a regular routine.

In terms of digestion, Vata individuals may experience irregular appetite and digestion, often leaning towards bloating, gas, and constipation. Their sensitivity to cold and dryness means they benefit from warm, nourishing foods and practices that promote relaxation and stability.

Balancing Vata involves countering its light, dry, and mobile nature with grounding, warming, and moisturizing influences. This can include eating warm, cooked foods, practicing regular routines, and engaging in calming activities like meditation and gentle yoga.

Pitta: The Energy of Transformation

Pitta is the dosha associated with the elements of Fire and Water. It governs all processes of transformation in the body, including digestion, metabolism, and the regulation of body temperature. Pitta is hot, sharp, light, and oily, and these qualities are evident in individuals with a Pitta-dominant constitution.

Those with a Pitta constitution typically have a medium build, a warm body temperature and often a reddish or yellowish complexion. They are known for their sharp intellect, strong willpower, and leadership abilities. However, when out of balance, Pitta can manifest as irritability, anger, and a tendency towards perfectionism.

Pitta individuals have a strong digestive fire, or Agni, which allows them to process food efficiently and maintain a steady appetite. However, they may also be prone to acidity, heartburn, and inflammatory conditions when Pitta is aggravated. Their natural heat makes them sensitive to hot weather, spicy foods, and competitive environments.

Balancing Pitta involves cooling, soothing, and calming influences to counter its fiery nature. This can be achieved through a diet that includes cooling foods like cucumbers, melons, and leafy greens, as well as engaging in relaxing activities that promote mental clarity and emotional balance.

Kapha: The Energy of Structure

Kapha is the dosha associated with the elements of Earth and Water, representing stability, structure, and cohesiveness in the body. It governs the formation of tissues, the storage of energy, and the body's immune system. Kapha is heavy, slow, steady, and moist, and these qualities are reflected in individuals with a Kapha-dominant constitution.

Individuals with a Kapha constitution tend to have a larger, more robust build, with smooth, oily skin and thick hair. They are often calm, patient, and nurturing, but may also struggle with lethargy, attachment, and resistance to change when out of balance. Kapha types have a steady and slow metabolism, which can make them prone to weight gain and fluid retention.

Kapha's grounding nature provides stability and endurance, but it can also lead to stagnation, both physically and mentally. When Kapha is imbalanced, it can manifest as sluggish digestion, congestion, and a tendency towards depression or emotional heaviness.

Balancing Kapha involves incorporating light, warming, and stimulating influences to counter its heavy and slow qualities. This can include eating light, spicy foods, engaging in regular exercise, and seeking out new experiences to break the cycle of inertia.

Dosha Imbalances and Health Implications

Symptoms and Causes of Imbalance

In Ayurveda, health is defined as a state of balance among the doshas. When one or more doshas become imbalanced, it can lead to physical, mental, and emotional disturbances. These imbalances are often caused by factors such as improper diet, stress, environmental influences, and seasonal changes.

- **Vata Imbalance:** When Vata is out of balance, its dry, light, and mobile qualities become excessive, leading to symptoms such as dryness of the skin and hair, constipation, bloating, and irregular menstrual cycles. Mentally, an aggravated Vata can cause anxiety, restlessness, and difficulty concentrating. Common causes of Vata imbalance include irregular eating habits, excessive travel, and exposure to cold, dry weather.

- **Pitta Imbalance:** Excess Pitta can result in the exacerbation of its hot and sharp qualities, leading to symptoms like acid reflux, ulcers, inflammation, and skin rashes. Emotionally, Pitta imbalance may manifest as anger, irritability, and impatience. Factors that contribute to Pitta imbalance include consuming spicy or acidic foods, exposure to hot weather, and high levels of stress or competition.

- **Kapha Imbalance:** When Kapha becomes excessive, its heavy and sluggish qualities dominate, causing symptoms such as weight gain, congestion, water retention, and lethargy. Mentally, a Kapha imbalance can lead to feelings of depression, attachment, and resistance to change. Causes of Kapha imbalance include overeating, lack of physical activity, and prolonged exposure to cold, damp environments.

Understanding the signs of dosha imbalances is crucial for early intervention and the prevention of more serious health issues. By recognizing these symptoms, you can take proactive steps to restore balance through dietary adjustments, lifestyle changes, and Ayurvedic treatments.

Effects on Physical and Mental Health

Dosha imbalances not only affect the physical body but also have a profound impact on mental and emotional health. Ayurveda teaches that the mind and body are intimately connected, and an imbalance in one can lead to disturbances in the other.

- **Vata and Mental Health:** An imbalanced Vata can cause feelings of fear, anxiety, and instability. The excessive movement and dryness associated with Vata can lead to a scattered mind, making it difficult to focus and make decisions. This mental agitation can also contribute to insomnia and other sleep disorders.

- **Pitta and Mental Health:** When Pitta is out of balance, it can lead to intense emotions such as anger, frustration, and jealousy. The fiery nature of Pitta can cause a person to become overly critical, competitive, and prone to burnout. Mental agitation from Pitta imbalance can also result in stress-related conditions such as hypertension and migraines.

- **Kapha and Mental Health:** A Kapha imbalance can manifest as mental stagnation, depression, and a lack of motivation. The heavy and stable qualities of Kapha, when excessive, can lead to a feeling of being "stuck" in life, with an inability to move forward or embrace change. This can result in emotional eating, withdrawal from social activities, and a general sense of apathy.

Balancing the doshas is key to maintaining not only physical health but also mental and emotional well-being. By addressing dosha imbalances, you can enhance your mental clarity, emotional resilience, and overall quality of life.

Determining Your Dosha

Self-Assessment Techniques

Determining your dosha is the first step in personalizing your Ayurvedic practice. There are several self-assessment techniques that can help you identify your dominant dosha and any imbalances that may be present.

One of the simplest methods is to take an Ayurvedic dosha quiz, which consists of a series of questions about your physical characteristics, personality traits, and habits. These quizzes are designed to help you identify which dosha is most predominant in your constitution.

In addition to quizzes, you can observe your body's natural tendencies, such as your digestive patterns, energy levels, and emotional responses. For example, if you have a strong, consistent appetite and tend to feel warm, you may have a dominant Pitta dosha. If you are more prone to cold hands and feet, irregular digestion, and frequent worry, Vata may be your predominant dosha.

It's also helpful to pay attention to the qualities of your skin, hair, and body type, as these can provide clues about your dosha. Vata types often have dry skin and thin hair, Pitta types may have sensitive or oily skin with fine hair, and Kapha types typically have smooth, oily skin and thick hair.

Professional Consultations

While self-assessment can provide valuable insights, a professional consultation with an Ayurvedic practitioner offers a more comprehensive understanding of your dosha constitution. Ayurvedic practitioners are trained to assess your Prakriti through various diagnostic methods, including pulse diagnosis, tongue analysis, and an in-depth discussion of your health history and lifestyle.

Pulse diagnosis, or Nadi Pariksha, is a key tool in Ayurveda for determining dosha balance. By feeling the radial pulse at the wrist, a practitioner can detect subtle variations in the pulse that correspond to the different doshas. This technique provides a deeper understanding of the current state of your doshas and any imbalances that may need to be addressed.

Tongue analysis, or Jihva Pariksha, involves examining the color, texture, and coating of the tongue, which can reveal information about your digestion, metabolism, and overall health. For example, a white coating on the tongue may indicate a Kapha imbalance, while a red or inflamed tongue could suggest excess Pitta.

During a consultation, the practitioner will also consider your mental and emotional state, as well as your diet, daily routines, and any symptoms you may be experiencing. This holistic assessment allows for a personalized treatment plan that addresses your unique needs and supports the balance of your doshas.

By combining self-assessment with professional guidance, you can gain a deeper understanding of your dosha constitution and how to maintain balance in your life. This knowledge empowers you to make informed decisions about your health and well-being, leading to a more harmonious and fulfilling life.

In this chapter, we have explored the three doshas—Vata, Pitta, and Kapha—their characteristics, and how they influence your physical, mental, and emotional health. Understanding the doshas is a crucial step in personalizing your Ayurvedic practice and achieving balance in your life. We also discussed the importance of recognizing and addressing dosha imbalances, as well as the methods for determining your unique dosha constitution.

As we move forward, the next chapter will delve into Ayurvedic nutrition and diet, exploring how you can use food as medicine to balance your doshas and support overall health. By tailoring your diet to your dosha constitution, you can optimize your digestion, boost your energy, and promote long-term wellness.

Chapter 3:
Ayurvedic Nutrition and Diet

In Ayurveda, diet is considered one of the most powerful tools for maintaining health and preventing disease. The food we eat not only nourishes our body but also has a profound impact on our mind, emotions, and overall well-being. Ayurveda views food as medicine, emphasizing the importance of choosing the right foods to balance the doshas and support optimal health. This chapter will explore the role of diet in Ayurveda, how to balance your doshas through food, and the importance of adjusting your diet according to seasonal changes and lifestyle needs. By understanding these principles, you can create a diet that promotes harmony, vitality, and longevity.

The Role of Diet in Ayurveda

Food as Medicine

In Ayurveda, food is not just a source of energy; it is also a form of medicine that can heal the body and mind. The ancient texts of Ayurveda emphasize the importance of a balanced diet as the foundation of good health. According to Ayurvedic principles, the quality of the food we consume directly affects our physical, mental, and spiritual well-being. Therefore, choosing the right foods is crucial for maintaining balance and preventing disease.

The concept of food as medicine in Ayurveda is based on the idea that different foods have specific qualities and effects on the body. These qualities, known as "gunas," can be categorized as heavy or light, hot or cold, dry or oily, and so on. Each food's qualities interact with the doshas in the body, either balancing or aggravating them. For example, heavy, oily foods may aggravate Kapha but pacify Vata, while light, cooling foods may pacify Pitta but aggravate Vata.

Ayurveda also recognizes the importance of digestion in the healing process. The digestive fire, or "Agni," is responsible for transforming food into energy and nutrients. When Agni is strong, the body can efficiently digest and assimilate food, leading to optimal health. However, when Agni is weak or imbalanced, It can result in the accumulation of toxins, known as "Ama," which can lead to disease. Therefore, Ayurveda places great emphasis on eating foods that support a strong and balanced digestive fire.

Principles of Ayurvedic Eating

Ayurveda offers several principles of eating that can help you maintain balance and support your overall health. These principles are designed to optimize digestion, enhance nutrient absorption, and prevent the accumulation of toxins in the body.

- **Eat According to Your Dosha:** One of the key principles of Ayurvedic eating is to choose foods that balance your dominant dosha. For example, if you have a Vata constitution, you may benefit from warm, nourishing foods that are grounding and easy to digest. Pitta individuals may thrive on cooling, hydrating foods that soothe their fiery nature, while Kapha types may need light, stimulating foods that counteract their natural heaviness.

- **Favor Fresh, Seasonal Foods:** Ayurveda emphasizes the importance of eating fresh, seasonal foods that are in harmony with the natural cycles of the environment. Seasonal foods are believed to be more nutritious and easier to digest, as they align with the body's changing needs throughout the year. For example, in the winter, you might favor warm, cooked foods that provide nourishment and warmth, while in the summer, you might choose cooling, hydrating foods that help you stay cool and refreshed.

- **Eat Mindfully:** Mindful eating is a central tenet of Ayurveda. This means eating with full awareness, savoring each bite, and paying attention to how your body responds to the food. Avoid distractions such as watching TV or using your phone while eating and take the time to chew your food thoroughly. Mindful eating not only enhances digestion but also helps you develop a deeper connection with your body and its needs.

- **Follow Regular Mealtimes:** Ayurveda recommends eating meals at regular intervals each day to support a stable digestive fire. Breakfast should be light and easy to digest, while lunch should be the largest meal of the day, eaten when Agni is at its peak. Dinner should be lighter and eaten a few hours before bedtime to allow for proper digestion before sleep.

- **Balance the Six Tastes:** Ayurveda identifies six tastes—sweet, sour, salty, bitter, pungent, and astringent—that should be included in each meal to create a balanced diet. Each taste has specific effects on the doshas and the body, and incorporating all six tastes helps ensure that your meals are nutritionally complete and satisfying. For example, sweet, sour, and salty tastes are grounding and nourishing, while bitter, pungent, and astringent tastes are cleansing and detoxifying.

By following these principles, you can create a diet that supports your unique constitution and promotes overall health and well-being.

Balancing Doshas through Diet

Vata-Pacifying Foods

Vata is characterized by the qualities of lightness, dryness, coldness, and mobility. When Vata is out of balance, it can lead to symptoms such as anxiety, restlessness, dry skin, and irregular digestion. To pacify Vata, it is important to choose foods that are warm, moist, and grounding.

- **Warm, Cooked Foods:** Vata types benefit from warm, cooked foods that are easy to digest. Soups, stews, and casseroles are ideal, as they provide both warmth and moisture. Avoid raw, cold foods such as salads and smoothies, which can aggravate Vata's cold and dry qualities.

- **Healthy Fats:** Incorporating healthy fats into the diet is essential for balancing Vata. Ghee (clarified butter), olive oil, and sesame oil are particularly nourishing for Vata. These fats help to lubricate the body, support digestion, and calm the nervous system.

- **Sweet and Sour Tastes:** The sweet and sour tastes are grounding and stabilizing for Vata. Sweet foods like root vegetables, grains, and dairy products provide nourishment and energy, while sour foods like citrus fruits and fermented foods stimulate digestion and enhance nutrient absorption.

- **Avoid Stimulants:** Vata types should avoid stimulants such as caffeine and alcohol, as these can increase anxiety and restlessness. Instead, opt for calming herbal teas such as chamomile, ashwagandha, or licorice root.

Pitta-Pacifying Foods

Pitta is characterized by the qualities of heat, sharpness, lightness, and intensity. When Pitta is out of balance, it can lead to symptoms such as inflammation, acidity, irritability, and skin rashes. To pacify Pitta, it is important to choose foods that are cooling, soothing, and hydrating.

- **Cooling Foods:** Pitta types benefit from cooling foods that help to counteract their natural heat. Fresh fruits and vegetables, particularly cucumbers, melons, leafy greens, and zucchini, are excellent choices. These foods provide hydration and help to reduce internal heat.

- **Bitter and Astringent Tastes:** The bitter and astringent tastes are particularly balancing for Pitta. Foods like leafy greens, cruciferous vegetables (such as broccoli and cauliflower), and legumes provide these tastes, which help to cleanse the body and reduce inflammation.

- **Sweet and Hydrating Foods:** Sweet and hydrating foods such as coconut, dairy products, and grains like rice and oats are soothing for Pitta. These foods help to cool the body and provide sustained energy without overheating the digestive system.

- **Avoid Spicy and Oily Foods:** Pitta types should avoid spicy, oily, and acidic foods, as these can aggravate their natural heat and lead to imbalances. Instead, opt for milder, cooling spices such as coriander, fennel, and mint.

Kapha-Pacifying Foods

Kapha is characterized by the qualities of heaviness, coldness, slowness, and stability. When Kapha is out of balance, it can lead to symptoms such as weight gain, congestion, sluggish digestion, and lethargy. To pacify

Kapha, it is important to choose foods that are light, warming, and stimulating.

- **Light and Dry Foods:** Kapha types benefit from light and dry foods that help to counteract their natural heaviness. Dry grains like quinoa, barley, and buckwheat are excellent choices, as they provide energy without adding excess moisture or heaviness to the body.

- **Warming Spices:** Incorporating warming spices into the diet is essential for balancing Kapha. Spices such as ginger, black pepper, turmeric, and cayenne pepper stimulate digestion, increase metabolism, and promote circulation.

- **Bitter, Pungent, and Astringent Tastes:** The bitter, pungent, and astringent tastes are particularly balancing for Kapha. Foods like leafy greens, radishes, and lentils provide these tastes, which help to detoxify the body and reduce stagnation.

- **Avoid Heavy and Oily Foods:** Kapha types should avoid heavy, oily, and sweet foods, as these can contribute to weight gain and sluggishness. Instead, focus on foods that are light, dry, and easy to digest.

By choosing foods that balance your dominant dosha, you can support your body's natural tendencies and promote optimal health.

Seasonal and Lifestyle Considerations

Adjusting Diet with Seasons

Ayurveda teaches that the changing seasons have a profound impact on our doshas and overall health. Each season brings with it different qualities that can either balance or aggravate the doshas, making it important to adjust your diet accordingly.

- **Winter (Vata Season):** During the winter, Vata's cold and dry qualities are heightened, making it important to focus on warm, nourishing foods. Root vegetables, whole grains, and healthy fats like ghee and sesame oil are ideal choices. Warm beverages like ginger tea can also help to keep Vata in balance.

- **Spring (Kapha Season):** In the spring, Kapha's heavy and sluggish qualities become more prominent, making it important to focus on light, cleansing foods. Leafy greens, sprouts, and bitter vegetables help to detoxify the body and reduce Kapha's excess. Incorporating warming spices like ginger and turmeric can also help to stimulate digestion and prevent congestion.

- **Summer (Pitta Season):** During the summer, Pitta's heat and intensity are at their peak, making it important to focus on cooling, hydrating foods. Fresh fruits and vegetables, particularly those with high water content, are ideal choices. Avoid spicy, oily foods that can aggravate Pitta and instead opt for cooling spices like coriander and mint.

- **Fall (Vata Season):** In the fall, Vata's cold and dry qualities return, making it important to focus on warm, grounding foods. Squash, sweet potatoes, and cooked grains are ideal choices. Adding warming spices like cinnamon and cardamom can also help to balance Vata and support digestion.

By adjusting your diet to align with the seasons, you can support your body's natural rhythms and maintain balance throughout the year.

Incorporating Ayurvedic Superfoods

Ayurveda also recognizes the importance of incorporating certain "superfoods" into the diet that provide exceptional nourishment and healing benefits. These foods are considered to be particularly balancing for the doshas and can be incorporated into your diet to enhance your overall health.

- **Turmeric:** Turmeric is a powerful anti-inflammatory spice that is particularly balancing for Pitta and Kapha doshas. It helps to cleanse the blood, reduce inflammation, and support healthy digestion. Turmeric can be added to a variety of dishes, including curries, soups, and smoothies, to boost its health benefits.

- **Ghee:** Ghee, or clarified butter, is considered a sacred and nourishing food in Ayurveda. It is particularly balancing for Vata and Pitta doshas, as it provides healthy fats that support digestion, lubrication, and mental clarity. Ghee can be used in cooking or as a topping for grains and vegetables.

- **Ashwagandha:** Ashwagandha is an adaptogenic herb that is particularly balancing for Vata and Kapha doshas. It helps to reduce stress, support the immune system, and promote overall vitality. Ashwagandha can be taken as a supplement or added to smoothies and teas.

- **Amalaki (Amla):** Amalaki, or Indian gooseberry, is a potent antioxidant and rejuvenating fruit that is particularly balancing for Pitta doshas. It helps to support digestion, boost immunity, and promote healthy skin and hair. Amalaki can be consumed as a juice, powder, or supplement.

- **Triphala:** Triphala is a traditional Ayurvedic formula made from three fruits: Amalaki, Bibhitaki, and Haritaki. It is particularly balancing for all three doshas and is known for its gentle detoxifying and rejuvenating effects. Triphala can be taken as a supplement or added to warm water as a digestive tonic.

Incorporating these Ayurvedic superfoods into your diet can provide additional support for balancing the doshas and promoting overall health and well-being.

In this chapter, we have explored the role of diet in Ayurveda, the principles of Ayurvedic eating, and how to balance your doshas through food. We also discussed the importance of adjusting your diet according to the seasons and incorporating Ayurvedic superfoods to enhance your overall health. By following these guidelines, you can create a diet that supports your unique constitution and promotes long-term wellness.

As we move forward, the next chapter will delve into the concept of Dinacharya, or daily routines, in Ayurveda. You will learn how to establish a balanced lifestyle by incorporating Ayurvedic practices into your daily routine, from morning rituals to evening wind-downs. These routines will help you maintain harmony in your body, mind, and spirit, supporting your journey to holistic well-being.

Chapter 4:
Daily Routines (Dinacharya)

In Ayurveda, Dinacharya, or daily routine, is considered one of the most powerful tools for maintaining balance and promoting health. The practice of Dinacharya involves aligning your daily activities with the natural rhythms of the day, ensuring that you support your body's innate intelligence and promote harmony in both body and mind. Establishing a consistent routine helps to stabilize the doshas, enhance digestion, and improve overall well-being. In this chapter, we will explore the importance of routine in Ayurveda, delve into specific morning and evening rituals, and discuss how these practices can support a balanced and fulfilling life.

The Importance of Routine

Establishing a Balanced Lifestyle

Ayurveda teaches that the human body is deeply connected to the cycles of nature, including the daily rhythms of the sun and moon. By aligning your daily activities with these natural rhythms, you can maintain balance and support optimal health. Establishing a daily routine, or Dinacharya, helps to regulate the body's internal clock, known as the circadian rhythm, which governs various physiological processes such as digestion, sleep, and hormone production.

A balanced lifestyle is one in which all aspects of life—physical, mental, emotional, and spiritual—are given due attention. This balance is essential for maintaining harmony among the doshas and preventing imbalances that can lead to disease. When your lifestyle is erratic or inconsistent, it can disrupt the natural flow of energy in the body, leading to disturbances in digestion, sleep, and mental clarity.

By establishing a daily routine, you create a stable foundation that supports your body's natural rhythms. This routine acts as an anchor, providing a sense of structure and stability that allows you to navigate the challenges of daily life with greater ease and resilience. Whether it's the time you wake up, the meals you eat, or the activities you engage in, consistency is key to maintaining balance and well-being.

Benefits of Consistent Practices

The benefits of maintaining a consistent daily routine are numerous and far-reaching. Some of the key benefits include:

- **Enhanced Digestion:** Regular meal times and consistent eating habits help to strengthen Agni, the digestive fire. When you eat at the same times each day, your body learns to anticipate and prepare for food, leading to more efficient digestion and nutrient absorption.

- **Improved Sleep Quality:** Following a regular sleep schedule helps to regulate the body's sleep-wake cycle, leading to better sleep quality and more restful nights. Going to bed and waking up at the same time each day supports the natural production of melatonin, the hormone that governs sleep.

- **Increased Energy Levels:** A consistent routine helps to regulate the body's energy levels, preventing the highs and lows that can occur with irregular habits. By aligning your activities with the natural rhythms of the day, you can optimize your energy levels and maintain vitality throughout the day.

- **Mental Clarity and Focus:** Regular routines help to calm the mind and reduce mental clutter, leading to greater clarity and focus. When you follow a consistent routine, your mind is less likely to be distracted by the unpredictability of the day, allowing you to concentrate on the tasks at hand.

- **Reduced Stress and Anxiety:** Consistency in daily practices helps to reduce stress and anxiety by providing a sense of predictability and control. When you know what to expect from your day, you are less likely to feel overwhelmed or anxious about the unknown.

- **Enhanced Emotional Stability:** A regular routine helps to stabilize the emotions, reducing mood swings and promoting a sense of calm and balance. By following consistent practices, you can create a stable emotional foundation that supports your overall well-being.

By incorporating these consistent practices into your daily routine, you can create a lifestyle that supports your physical, mental, and emotional health, leading to a more balanced and fulfilling life.

Morning Rituals

Tongue Scraping and Oil Pulling

The morning is a time of renewal and rejuvenation, and Ayurveda places great importance on starting the day with practices that cleanse and nourish the body. Two key morning rituals in Ayurveda are tongue scraping and oil pulling, both of which are designed to support oral health and overall well-being.

- **Tongue Scraping:** Tongue scraping is a simple yet powerful practice that involves using a metal scraper to gently remove the coating that forms on the tongue overnight. This coating, known as "Ama," is a buildup of toxins that can accumulate in the body as a result of poor digestion, stress, or imbalanced doshas. By removing this coating first thing in the morning, you help to eliminate toxins from the body and prevent them from being reabsorbed.

Tongue scraping also stimulates the taste buds, which in turn activates the digestive system and prepares it for the day's meals. It enhances the sense of taste, allowing you to fully enjoy the flavors of your food, and can also help to reduce bad breath and improve oral hygiene. To practice tongue scraping, simply use a metal tongue scraper (preferably made of copper or stainless steel) and gently scrape the surface of the tongue from back to front, rinsing the scraper after each pass.

- **Oil Pulling:** Oil pulling is an ancient Ayurvedic practice that involves swishing oil (typically sesame or coconut oil) in the mouth for several minutes to cleanse the oral cavity and promote overall health. The oil acts as a natural detoxifier, drawing out toxins, bacteria, and debris from the mouth and gums.

Oil pulling is believed to support oral health by reducing plaque buildup, preventing cavities, and promoting healthy gums. It can also help to whiten teeth and freshen breath. In addition to its oral health benefits, oil pulling is said to have a balancing effect on the doshas, particularly Vata and Kapha, by lubricating the tissues and calming the nervous system.

To practice oil pulling, take a tablespoon of oil and swish it around in your mouth for 15-20 minutes, making sure to move the oil through all areas of the mouth. After swishing, spit the oil out into a trash bin (avoid spitting it into the sink to prevent clogging) and rinse your mouth with warm water. Follow this practice with tooth brushing and tongue scraping for a complete oral hygiene routine.

Abhyanga (Self-Massage)

Abhyanga, or self-massage, is a deeply nourishing and rejuvenating practice that involves applying warm oil to the entire body. This practice is particularly balancing for Vata dosha, but it can be beneficial for all doshas when practiced regularly. Abhyanga helps to nourish the skin, calm the nervous system, and promote overall well-being.

- **The Benefits of Abhyanga:** Abhyanga offers numerous benefits for the body and mind. The application of warm oil helps to lubricate the joints, improve circulation, and promote flexibility. It also nourishes the skin, leaving it soft and supple, while helping to remove toxins from the body. The gentle pressure and rhythmic movements of the massage have a calming effect on the nervous system, reducing stress and anxiety.

In addition to its physical benefits, Abhyanga is a deeply grounding practice that helps to balance the doshas, particularly Vata. The practice of self-massage can also enhance body awareness, promoting a deeper connection with your physical self and fostering a sense of self-love and care.

- **How to Perform Abhyanga:** To perform Abhyanga, start by warming a small amount of oil (sesame oil is recommended for Vata, coconut oil for Pitta, and mustard or olive oil for Kapha) in a double boiler or by placing the bottle of oil in hot water. Once the oil is warm, begin the massage by applying the oil to your scalp and face, using gentle circular motions. Move on to the neck, shoulders, and arms, using long strokes on the limbs and circular motions on the joints. Continue to massage the abdomen and chest in clockwise circular motions, followed by long strokes on the back and sides of the torso.

Finish the massage by applying oil to the legs, using long strokes on the limbs and circular motions on the joints. Take your time with the massage, allowing yourself to fully relax and enjoy the experience. After the massage, allow the oil to absorb into the skin for 15-20 minutes before taking a warm shower or bath.

Incorporating Abhyanga into your morning routine can help to set a positive tone for the day, leaving you feeling nourished, grounded, and ready to face whatever challenges come your way.

Evening Rituals

Winding Down Techniques

Just as the morning is a time for renewal, the evening is a time for winding down and preparing the body and mind for restful sleep. Ayurveda emphasizes the importance of creating a calming evening routine that helps to release the stresses of the day and promote relaxation. By incorporating specific winding-down techniques into your evening routine, you can support the transition from wakefulness to sleep and enhance the quality of your rest.

- **Creating a Calming Environment:** The environment in which you spend your evening has a significant impact on your ability to relax and unwind. Ayurveda recommends creating a calming environment by dimming the lights, reducing noise, and avoiding stimulating activities such as watching TV or using electronic devices. Instead, opt for activities that promote relaxation, such as reading, journaling, or listening to soothing music.

- **Practicing Gentle Yoga or Stretching:** Gentle yoga or stretching exercises can help to release tension from the body and calm the mind. Poses such as forward bends, gentle twists, and restorative postures are particularly effective for promoting relaxation and preparing the body for sleep. Practicing a few minutes of gentle yoga before bed can help to ease muscle tension, improve circulation, and promote a sense of calm.

- **Aromatherapy for Relaxation:** Aromatherapy is a powerful tool for promoting relaxation and enhancing the quality of sleep. Essential oils such as lavender, chamomile, and sandalwood have calming properties that can help to reduce stress and anxiety. You can incorporate aromatherapy into your evening routine by using a diffuser, applying essential oils to your pulse points, or adding a few drops of oil to your bath.

Promoting Restful Sleep

Getting a good night's sleep is essential for maintaining balance and overall health. Ayurveda recognizes the importance of sleep as one of the three pillars of life, along with diet and lifestyle. To promote restful sleep, it is important to follow a consistent bedtime routine that helps to calm the mind and prepare the body for rest.

- **Establish a Regular Sleep Schedule:** Ayurveda recommends going to bed and waking up at the same time each day to regulate the body's sleep-wake cycle. Aim to go to bed by 10:00 PM, as this is the time when the body naturally begins to wind down and prepare for sleep. Waking up early, around 6:00

AM, allows you to align with the natural rhythms of the day and start your morning routine with energy and clarity.

- **Practice Pranayama or Meditation:** Pranayama (breathing exercises) and meditation are powerful tools for calming the mind and promoting relaxation. Practices such as deep belly breathing, alternate nostril breathing, or simple mindfulness meditation can help to reduce mental chatter, release stress, and prepare the mind for sleep. Incorporating these practices into your evening routine can enhance the quality of your sleep and support overall well-being.

- **Herbal Remedies for Sleep:** Ayurveda offers several herbal remedies that can help to promote restful sleep. Herbs such as ashwagandha, valerian, and brahmi are known for their calming and sedative properties. You can take these herbs as a supplement, in the form of a tea, or as part of an Ayurvedic formula designed to support sleep. Drinking a cup of warm milk with a pinch of nutmeg before bed is another traditional Ayurvedic remedy for promoting restful sleep.

By following these evening rituals, you can create a bedtime routine that supports deep, restful sleep and enhances your overall health and well-being.

In this chapter, we have explored the importance of daily routines, or Dinacharya, in Ayurveda. We discussed the benefits of establishing a consistent routine, as well as specific morning and evening rituals that can help you maintain balance and promote overall health. By incorporating these practices into your daily life, you can create a stable foundation that supports your physical, mental, and emotional well-being.

As we move forward, the next chapter will delve into the use of Ayurvedic herbal remedies, exploring how you can incorporate herbs into your daily routine to support your health and balance your doshas. These remedies will provide additional tools to enhance your well-being and promote long-term vitality.

Chapter 5:
Ayurvedic Herbal Remedies

Ayurveda has long recognized the powerful healing properties of herbs, viewing them as essential components of a holistic approach to health and wellness. Ayurvedic herbs are used to balance the doshas, support the body's natural healing processes, and promote overall vitality. This chapter will introduce you to the foundational concepts of Ayurvedic herbalism, explore some of the most revered Ayurvedic herbs and their uses, and guide you through the process of making your own herbal preparations. By understanding the role of herbs in Ayurveda, you can incorporate these natural remedies into your daily routine to enhance your well-being and achieve greater harmony in your life.

Introduction to Ayurvedic Herbs

Understanding Herbal Properties

In Ayurveda, herbs are classified according to their qualities, or "gunas," which describe the effects they have on the body and mind. These qualities are used to determine how an herb interacts with the doshas and which imbalances it can help to correct. The gunas of an herb may include its temperature (hot or cold), its moisture level (dry or oily), its heaviness (light or heavy), and its potency (mild or strong).

Each herb also has a specific taste, or "rasa," which plays a crucial role in its therapeutic action. Ayurveda identifies six primary tastes: sweet, sour, salty, bitter, pungent, and astringent. Each taste has specific effects on the doshas, with some tastes balancing certain doshas while aggravating others. For example, sweet and cooling herbs are often used to pacify Pitta, while warming and stimulating herbs are used to balance Kapha.

In addition to their physical properties, Ayurvedic herbs are believed to possess "virya" (potency) and "vipaka" (post-digestive effect), which influence their long-term impact on the body. The virya of an herb refers to its immediate effect after consumption, such as heating or cooling, while the vipaka describes the herb's effect after digestion, which can be either sweet, sour, or pungent.

Understanding these herbal properties is essential for selecting the right herbs to address specific health concerns and dosha imbalances. Ayurvedic practitioners use this knowledge to create personalized herbal remedies that align with an individual's unique constitution and health needs.

Sourcing and Quality Considerations

The effectiveness of Ayurvedic herbs depends not only on their properties but also on their quality. High-quality herbs are grown, harvested, and processed with care to preserve their potency and therapeutic benefits. When sourcing Ayurvedic herbs, it is important to consider factors such as the origin of the herbs, the farming practices used, and the processing methods employed.

- **Organic and Sustainable Farming:** Ayurvedic herbs should be grown using organic and sustainable farming practices to ensure that they are free from pesticides, herbicides, and other harmful chemicals. Organic farming also supports the health of the soil, which in turn enhances the nutritional value and potency of the herbs.

- **Ethical Harvesting:** Herbs should be harvested at the optimal time, when their active compounds are at their peak. Ethical harvesting practices ensure that the plants are not over-harvested or damaged, allowing them to continue thriving in their natural environment. This is especially important for wild-harvested herbs, which may be at risk of depletion if not harvested responsibly.

- **Proper Processing:** The processing of Ayurvedic herbs plays a crucial role in preserving their potency. Herbs should be dried, powdered, and stored in a way that protects them from exposure to light, heat, and moisture. Some herbs may also undergo additional processing, such as decoction or fermentation, to enhance their therapeutic properties.

When purchasing Ayurvedic herbs, it is important to choose reputable suppliers who prioritize quality and sustainability. Look for certifications such as organic, fair trade, and non-GMO, and inquire about the sourcing and processing methods used. By choosing high-quality herbs, you can ensure that you are receiving the full benefits of these powerful natural remedies.

Top Ayurvedic Herbs and Their Uses

Ashwagandha, Turmeric, and Triphala

Ayurveda has a vast pharmacopeia of herbs, each with its unique properties and therapeutic benefits. In this section, we will explore three of the most revered Ayurvedic herbs—Ashwagandha, Turmeric, and Triphala—and how they can be used to support health and balance the doshas.

- **Ashwagandha (Withania somnifera):** Ashwagandha, also known as "Indian ginseng" or "winter cherry," is a powerful adaptogenic herb that is highly valued in Ayurveda for its ability to enhance vitality and resilience. Ashwagandha is particularly balancing for Vata and Kapha doshas, though it can be beneficial for all doshas when used appropriately.

    Ashwagandha is known for its ability to reduce stress and anxiety, support the immune system, and promote restful sleep. It is also used to improve energy levels, stamina, and cognitive function. In addition to its adaptogenic properties, Ashwagandha has anti-inflammatory and antioxidant effects, making it useful for managing chronic conditions such as arthritis and inflammation.

Ashwagandha can be taken in various forms, including as a powder, capsule, or tincture. It is often combined with other herbs to enhance its effects. For example, it may be mixed with warm milk and honey to promote relaxation and restful sleep or added to a rejuvenating herbal blend to support overall vitality.

- **Turmeric (Curcuma longa):** Turmeric is one of the most well-known and widely used herbs in Ayurveda, prized for its powerful anti-inflammatory, antioxidant, and healing properties. Turmeric is particularly balancing for Pitta and Kapha doshas, though it can be beneficial for Vata dosha in moderation.

  The active compound in turmeric, curcumin, is responsible for many of its therapeutic effects. Turmeric is commonly used to support digestion, reduce inflammation, and promote healthy skin. It is also used to support liver function, enhance immunity, and protect against oxidative stress.

  Turmeric can be incorporated into the diet as a spice, added to teas or golden milk, or taken as a supplement in capsule or powder form. It is often combined with black pepper, which enhances the bioavailability of curcumin and increases its effectiveness. Turmeric can also be applied topically as a paste to treat skin conditions or wounds.

- **Triphala:** Triphala is a traditional Ayurvedic formula composed of three fruits: Amalaki (Emblica officinalis),

Bibhitaki (Terminalia bellirica), and Haritaki (Terminalia chebula). This powerful combination is known for its gentle detoxifying and rejuvenating effects and is considered one of the most important herbal formulations in Ayurveda. Triphala is balancing for all three doshas and is particularly valued for its ability to support digestion, detoxification, and overall health.

Triphala is commonly used to promote regular bowel movements, improve digestion, and cleanse the colon. It also has antioxidant properties, supporting the body's natural detoxification processes and protecting against free radical damage. In addition to its digestive benefits, Triphala is used to support eye health, enhance immunity, and promote longevity.

Triphala can be taken as a powder, capsule, or tea. It is typically consumed in the evening before bed to support overnight detoxification and promote regularity. The powder can be mixed with warm water or honey, while the capsules offer a convenient option for those who prefer a more straightforward method of consumption.

Herbal Blends and Formulas

In addition to individual herbs, Ayurveda makes extensive use of herbal blends and formulas, which combine multiple herbs to enhance their synergistic effects. These blends are often designed to target specific health concerns or dosha imbalances and are tailored to the individual's unique constitution and needs.

- **Chyawanprash:** Chyawanprash is a traditional Ayurvedic herbal jam made from a blend of herbs, fruits, and spices, with Amalaki as the primary

ingredient. It is a powerful rejuvenative tonic that is particularly beneficial for boosting immunity, enhancing vitality, and promoting overall health. Chyawanprash is balancing for all doshas and can be taken daily as a health supplement.
- **Trikatu:** Trikatu is a warming herbal blend made from three pungent spices: black pepper, long pepper (Pippali), and ginger. This formula is particularly balancing for Kapha and Vata doshas and is used to stimulate digestion, enhance metabolism, and support respiratory health. Trikatu can be taken before meals to improve digestion or used as a spice in cooking.
- **Dashamoola:** Dashamoola is a traditional Ayurvedic formula made from the roots of ten different herbs. It is particularly valued for its anti-inflammatory and analgesic properties and is used to support joint and muscle health, relieve pain, and promote overall balance. Dashamoola is balancing for Vata dosha and can be taken as a decoction, powder, or capsule.
- **Brahmi Ghrita:** Brahmi Ghrita is a traditional Ayurvedic ghee (clarified butter) infused with Brahmi (Bacopa monnieri) and other herbs. It is particularly valued for its ability to enhance cognitive function, support mental clarity, and promote relaxation. Brahmi Ghrita is balancing for Vata and Pitta doshas and can be taken as a supplement or used as a cooking oil.

These herbal blends and formulas offer a convenient and effective way to incorporate the benefits of multiple herbs into your daily routine. By using these time-honored preparations, you can support your health and well-being in a holistic and balanced way.

Making Herbal Preparations

Teas, Tinctures, and Powders

One of the strengths of Ayurveda is its practical approach to herbal medicine, which includes a variety of methods for preparing and consuming herbs. These methods allow you to tailor your herbal remedies to your specific needs and preferences.

- **Teas:** Herbal teas, or infusions, are one of the simplest and most effective ways to consume Ayurvedic herbs. Teas are made by steeping dried or fresh herbs in hot water, allowing their active compounds to be extracted. Herbal teas can be made from single herbs or a blend of herbs, depending on the desired effect. For example, a calming tea made from chamomile, ashwagandha, and licorice root can help to reduce stress and promote relaxation.

- **Tinctures:** Tinctures are concentrated herbal extracts made by soaking herbs in alcohol or glycerin. This method extracts the active compounds from the herbs and preserves them in liquid form, making tinctures a convenient and potent way to consume herbs. Tinctures are typically taken in small doses, such as a few drops in water or under the tongue. They are particularly useful for herbs that are not easily extracted in water, such as roots and barks.

- **Powders:** Herbal powders are made by drying and finely grinding herbs into a powder form. Powders can be taken on their own, mixed with water, milk, or honey, or added to smoothies and other foods. Ayurvedic powders, such as Ashwagandha, Triphala, and Turmeric, are versatile and can be used in a variety of ways to support health and balance.

Dosage and Safety Guidelines

While Ayurvedic herbs are generally considered safe when used appropriately, it is important to follow proper dosage guidelines to avoid potential side effects or interactions. The correct dosage of an herb depends on several factors, including the individual's constitution, the specific health concern being addressed, and the form in which the herb is consumed.

- **General Dosage Guidelines:** For most Ayurvedic herbs, the typical dosage ranges from 500 mg to 1 gram per day for powders and capsules, or 1-2 teaspoons per day for teas and tinctures. However, some herbs may require higher or lower doses depending on their potency and intended use. It is always best to start with a lower dose and gradually increase it as needed, while monitoring your body's response.

- **Consulting a Practitioner:** If you are new to Ayurvedic herbs or have specific health concerns, it is advisable to consult with a qualified Ayurvedic practitioner before starting any herbal regimen. A practitioner can provide personalized guidance on the appropriate herbs, dosages, and preparations for your individual needs.

- **Safety Considerations:** Some Ayurvedic herbs may interact with medications or have contraindications for certain health conditions. For example, Turmeric, while generally safe, may interact with blood-thinning medications, and Ashwagandha should be used with caution in individuals with thyroid disorders. Pregnant and breastfeeding women should also consult with a healthcare provider before using Ayurvedic herbs.

By following these dosage and safety guidelines, you can ensure that you are using Ayurvedic herbs effectively and safely to support your health and well-being.

In this chapter, we have explored the rich tradition of Ayurvedic herbal remedies, from understanding the properties of herbs to sourcing high-quality ingredients and making your own preparations. We also discussed the therapeutic benefits of some of the most revered Ayurvedic herbs, including Ashwagandha, Turmeric, and Triphala, as well as the use of herbal blends and formulas to address specific health concerns.

As we move forward, the next chapter will delve into the role of meditation and yoga in Ayurveda, exploring how these practices can be integrated into your daily routine to support mental clarity, emotional balance, and overall well-being. By combining the power of herbs with the practices of meditation and yoga, you can create a holistic approach to health that nurtures both body and mind.

Chapter 6:
The Role of Meditation and Yoga

In Ayurveda, the mind and body are seen as interconnected, with each influencing the health and well-being of the other. Meditation and yoga are central practices in Ayurveda that help to balance the mind, strengthen the body, and promote harmony between the two. These practices are not just about physical exercise or mental relaxation; they are holistic tools that address the root causes of imbalance, enhancing overall health and well-being. In this chapter, we will explore the importance of the mind-body connection in Ayurveda, introduce Ayurvedic meditation techniques, and discuss how yoga can be tailored to balance the doshas. By incorporating these practices into your daily life, you can create a more balanced and fulfilling lifestyle.

Mind-Body Connection in Ayurveda

Benefits of Meditation and Yoga

Ayurveda views the mind and body as deeply interconnected, with the state of one affecting the other. When the mind is calm and clear, the body is more likely to be in a state of balance, and when the body is healthy, the mind is more likely to experience peace and clarity. This holistic perspective is the foundation for the integration of meditation and yoga into Ayurvedic practices.

- **Stress Reduction:** One of the primary benefits of meditation and yoga is their ability to reduce stress. Stress is a major contributor to dosha imbalances and can manifest as physical, mental, and emotional disturbances. Regular meditation helps to calm the mind, reduce anxiety, and promote a sense of inner peace, while yoga helps to release physical tension and enhance the body's resilience to stress.

- **Improved Mental Clarity:** Meditation and yoga enhance mental clarity and focus by quieting the mind and bringing attention to the present moment. This mindfulness allows for better decision-making, increased creativity, and a deeper understanding of oneself. By cultivating a calm and clear mind, you can improve your ability to navigate life's challenges with grace and wisdom.

- **Enhanced Physical Health:** Yoga, in particular, offers numerous physical benefits, including increased flexibility, strength, and balance. The physical postures, or asanas, help to improve circulation, support the health of the organs, and enhance the functioning of the respiratory and digestive systems. When combined with meditation, these practices also support the body's natural healing processes, promoting overall health and vitality.

- **Emotional Balance:** Meditation and yoga help to regulate emotions by calming the nervous system and promoting the release of feel-good hormones such as serotonin and dopamine. These practices can help to reduce mood swings, alleviate symptoms of depression and anxiety, and foster a greater sense of emotional stability and well-being.

- **Spiritual Growth:** In addition to their physical and mental benefits, meditation and yoga are powerful tools for spiritual growth. These practices help to quiet the mind, open the heart, and connect with a deeper sense of purpose and meaning. By cultivating a regular meditation and yoga practice, you can enhance your spiritual awareness and deepen your connection to the self and the world around you.

Incorporating Practices into Daily Life

Incorporating meditation and yoga into your daily routine does not require a significant time commitment. Even a few minutes of practice each day can have a profound impact on your well-being. The key is to approach these practices with consistency and intention, allowing them to become a regular part of your daily life.

- **Start with Small Steps:** If you are new to meditation and yoga, start with small, manageable steps. Begin with a short meditation session of 5-10 minutes each morning, or incorporate a few simple yoga poses into your morning routine. As you become more comfortable with these practices, you can gradually increase the duration and complexity of your sessions.

- **Create a Dedicated Space:** Designate a quiet and comfortable space in your home for meditation and yoga. This space should be free from distractions and clutter, allowing you to focus fully on your practice. Consider adding elements that promote relaxation, such as candles, incense, or soothing music.

- **Set a Consistent Schedule:** Consistency is key to reaping the benefits of meditation and yoga. Set aside a specific time each day for your practice, whether it's in the morning, during a lunch break, or before bed. By establishing a regular schedule, you create a routine that supports your physical, mental, and emotional well-being.

- **Listen to Your Body:** Both meditation and yoga should be approached with mindfulness and self-awareness. Listen to your body and mind, and adjust your practice as needed to meet your current needs. If you feel fatigued, opt for a gentler yoga session or a restorative meditation practice. If you have more energy, challenge yourself with a more vigorous yoga flow or a longer meditation session.

By incorporating meditation and yoga into your daily life, you can create a foundation for lasting health, balance, and well-being.

Ayurvedic Meditation Techniques

Guided Meditation and Mindfulness

Meditation is a central practice in Ayurveda, used to calm the mind, balance the doshas, and promote overall well-being. There are many different meditation techniques, but two of the most commonly used in Ayurveda are guided meditation and mindfulness meditation.

- **Guided Meditation:** Guided meditation involves listening to a recorded or live guide who leads you through a specific meditation practice. This can include visualization, body scans, or breath awareness exercises. Guided meditation is particularly helpful for beginners or those who struggle with maintaining focus during meditation, as the guide provides structure and direction throughout the practice.

    Guided meditations can be tailored to address specific needs, such as reducing stress, enhancing sleep, or cultivating self-compassion. For example, a guided meditation for stress relief might lead you through a visualization of a peaceful place, helping to calm the mind and release tension. A guided meditation for self-compassion might involve repeating affirmations or focusing on feelings of love and kindness.

- **Mindfulness Meditation:** Mindfulness meditation involves bringing your full attention to the present moment, without judgment or attachment. This practice helps to cultivate awareness and acceptance of your thoughts, emotions, and physical sensations, allowing you to observe them without becoming overwhelmed or reactive.

In mindfulness meditation, you can focus on your breath, a specific sensation in your body, or a mantra. The goal is not to clear your mind of thoughts but to observe them as they arise and pass, maintaining a state of non-attachment and equanimity. This practice helps to reduce mental clutter, improve focus, and enhance emotional resilience.

Both guided meditation and mindfulness meditation can be practiced for as little as 5-10 minutes a day, making them accessible to anyone, regardless of experience level. These practices can be used individually or combined, depending on your needs and preferences.

Pranayama (Breathing Exercises)

Pranayama, or breath control, is a powerful practice in Ayurveda that involves regulating the breath to influence the flow of energy, or "prana," within the body. Pranayama helps to balance the doshas, calm the mind, and enhance physical and mental health. There are several different pranayama techniques, each with its specific benefits.

- **Nadi Shodhana (Alternate Nostril Breathing):** Nadi Shodhana is a calming and balancing pranayama technique that involves alternating the breath between the left and right nostrils. This practice helps to balance the energy channels, or nadis, in the body, promoting mental clarity, emotional stability, and overall balance. Nadi Shodhana is particularly beneficial for balancing Vata dosha, as it helps to calm the nervous system and reduce anxiety.

    To practice Nadi Shodhana, sit comfortably with your spine straight. Close your right nostril with your right thumb and inhale deeply through your left nostril.

Then close your left nostril with your right ring finger, release your right nostril, and exhale through your right nostril. Inhale through your right nostril, then close it and exhale through your left nostril. Continue alternating for several rounds, focusing on your breath and the calming effects of the practice.

- **Kapalabhati (Skull-Shining Breath):** Kapalabhati is an energizing pranayama technique that involves short, forceful exhales followed by passive inhales. This practice helps to stimulate digestion, increase energy levels, and clear the mind. Kapalabhati is particularly balancing for Kapha dosha, as it helps to reduce stagnation and increase metabolism.

To practice Kapalabhati, sit comfortably with your spine straight. Take a deep inhale, then begin short, forceful exhales through your nose, contracting your abdominal muscles with each exhale. Allow the inhales to happen passively between each exhale. Continue for several rounds, then take a deep breath in and exhale slowly.

- **Bhramari (Bee Breath):** Bhramari is a calming pranayama technique that involves producing a humming sound during exhalation. This practice helps to soothe the nervous system, reduce stress, and promote relaxation. Bhramari is particularly balancing for Pitta dosha, as it helps to cool the mind and release tension.

To practice Bhramari, sit comfortably with your spine straight. Close your eyes and take a deep inhale. As you exhale, produce a humming sound, similar to the buzzing of a bee. Focus on the vibrations of the sound as it resonates through your body. Continue for several rounds, then sit quietly and observe the calming effects of the practice.

Pranayama can be practiced on its own or as part of a larger meditation or yoga routine. By incorporating pranayama into your daily practice, you can enhance your breath awareness, balance your energy, and support overall health and well-being.

Yoga for Dosha Balance

Vata, Pitta, and Kapha Yoga Practices

In Ayurveda, yoga is not a one-size-fits-all practice. Different yoga practices are recommended for different dosha types to help balance their unique qualities and tendencies. By tailoring your yoga practice to your dosha, you can enhance the benefits of the practice and promote greater balance in your life.

- **Vata Yoga:** Vata types tend to be naturally energetic and creative, but they can also be prone to anxiety, restlessness, and irregularity. To balance Vata, it is important to focus on grounding, calming, and stabilizing yoga practices. Slow, gentle movements, deep breathing, and restorative poses are particularly beneficial for Vata.

  A Vata-balancing yoga practice might include poses such as Mountain Pose (Tadasana), Tree Pose (Vrksasana), Child's Pose (Balasana), and Legs Up the Wall (Viparita Karani). These poses help to ground the energy, calm the mind, and promote a sense of stability and relaxation.

- **Pitta Yoga:** Pitta types are naturally focused, driven, and competitive, but they can also be prone to irritability, anger, and inflammation. To balance Pitta, it is important to focus on cooling, calming, and non-competitive yoga practices. Gentle flows, moderate intensity, and a focus on mindfulness are particularly beneficial for Pitta.

  A Pitta-balancing yoga practice might include poses such as Forward Fold (Uttanasana), Seated Forward Bend (Paschimottanasana), Cobra Pose (Bhujangasana), and Savasana (Corpse Pose). These poses help to release heat, calm the mind, and promote a sense of peace and relaxation.

- **Kapha Yoga:** Kapha types are naturally steady, strong, and nurturing, but they can also be prone to lethargy, stagnation, and attachment. To balance Kapha, it is important to focus on invigorating, stimulating, and energizing yoga practices. Dynamic flows, vigorous movements, and a focus on breathwork are particularly beneficial for Kapha.

  A Kapha-balancing yoga practice might include poses such as Sun Salutations (Surya Namaskar), Warrior Poses (Virabhadrasana I, II, III), Chair Pose (Utkatasana), and Bridge Pose (Setu Bandhasana). These poses help to increase energy, stimulate circulation, and promote a sense of lightness and vitality.

Customizing Your Yoga Routine

In addition to tailoring your yoga practice to your dosha, it is important to customize your routine based on your individual needs, preferences, and current state of balance.

This may involve adjusting the intensity, duration, and focus of your practice to align with your current physical, mental, and emotional state.

- **Listen to Your Body:** Your body is your best guide when it comes to customizing your yoga routine. Pay attention to how you feel before, during, and after your practice, and adjust accordingly. If you feel fatigued or overwhelmed, opt for a gentler practice. If you feel energized and motivated, challenge yourself with a more vigorous routine.

- **Incorporate Mindfulness:** Mindfulness is a key component of a customized yoga practice. By bringing your full attention to each movement, breath, and sensation, you can deepen your awareness of your body and mind, allowing you to make adjustments that support your overall well-being.

- **Adapt to the Seasons:** Just as you adjust your diet with the changing seasons, you can also adapt your yoga practice to align with seasonal shifts. In the winter, focus on warming and grounding practices to counteract the cold and dryness of Vata season. In the summer, focus on cooling and calming practices to balance the heat of Pitta season. In the spring, focus on invigorating and detoxifying practices to clear the stagnation of Kapha season.

By customizing your yoga routine, you can create a practice that is deeply aligned with your unique constitution, needs, and goals, enhancing the overall benefits of your practice.

In this chapter, we have explored the powerful role of meditation and yoga in Ayurveda, highlighting their benefits for the mind, body, and spirit. We discussed the importance of the mind-body connection, introduced Ayurvedic meditation techniques, and provided guidance on tailoring yoga practices to balance the doshas. By incorporating these practices into your daily routine, you can create a holistic approach to health and well-being that nurtures both body and mind.

As we move forward, the next chapter will delve into Ayurvedic detoxification, specifically focusing on Panchakarma, the traditional Ayurvedic cleansing process. You will learn about the importance of detoxification, the key procedures involved, and how to integrate these practices into your life for long-term health and vitality.

Chapter 7: Ayurvedic Detoxification (Panchakarma)

In Ayurveda, detoxification is considered an essential practice for maintaining balance and promoting overall health. The accumulation of toxins, or "Ama," in the body is believed to be the root cause of many diseases and imbalances. Regular detoxification helps to remove these toxins, restore the body's natural balance, and support optimal functioning of the mind, body, and spirit. Panchakarma, the traditional Ayurvedic detoxification process, is a comprehensive and powerful method for cleansing the body at a deep level. In this chapter, we will explore the need for detoxification, introduce the principles and procedures of Panchakarma, and provide guidance on at-home detox practices that can support long-term health.

The Need for Detoxification

Signs You Need a Detox

In Ayurveda, the accumulation of Ama, or toxins, is seen as a major contributor to imbalances and disease. Ama is created when the digestive fire, or "Agni," is weak or impaired, leading to incomplete digestion and the formation of toxic byproducts. These toxins can accumulate in the body, leading to physical, mental, and emotional disturbances.

There are several signs that indicate the presence of Ama in the body and the need for detoxification:

- **Digestive Issues:** Common signs of Ama include poor digestion, bloating, gas, constipation, or diarrhea. These symptoms suggest that the digestive system is not functioning optimally, leading to the buildup of toxins.

- **Fatigue and Lethargy:** If you frequently feel tired, sluggish, or lacking in energy, it may be a sign that your body is weighed down by toxins. Ama can interfere with the body's ability to produce and utilize energy, leading to chronic fatigue.

- **Mental Fog and Lack of Clarity:** Ama can also affect the mind, leading to mental fog, difficulty concentrating, and a lack of clarity. If you find it challenging to focus or make decisions, it may be time for a detox.

- **Skin Issues:** The skin is one of the body's primary detoxification organs, and when toxins accumulate, it can manifest as skin problems such as acne, rashes, or dullness. These symptoms may indicate that your body is struggling to eliminate toxins through the skin.

- **Bad Breath and Coated Tongue:** A thick coating on the tongue, particularly in the morning, is a classic sign of Ama. Bad breath, a sour or metallic taste in the mouth, and a coated tongue all suggest that toxins are present in the digestive system.

- **Joint and Muscle Pain:** Ama can accumulate in the joints and muscles, leading to stiffness, pain, and inflammation. If you experience frequent aches and pains without a clear cause, detoxification may help to relieve these symptoms.

- **Emotional Imbalance:** Ama can also affect the emotions, leading to feelings of irritability, anxiety, depression, or mood swings. Detoxification can help to clear these emotional toxins, promoting greater emotional stability and well-being.

If you recognize any of these signs in yourself, it may be time to consider a detox. Detoxification can help to remove Ama from the body, restore balance, and support overall health.

Benefits of Regular Detox

Regular detoxification offers numerous benefits for the mind, body, and spirit. By removing toxins and restoring balance, detoxification can enhance your overall well-being and prevent the onset of disease. Some of the key benefits of regular detox include:

- **Improved Digestion:** Detoxification helps to strengthen the digestive fire, or Agni, allowing your body to digest food more efficiently and absorb nutrients more effectively. This can lead to reduced bloating, gas, and constipation, as well as improved overall digestion.

- **Increased Energy Levels:** By removing toxins from the body, detoxification can help to restore your energy levels and reduce feelings of fatigue and lethargy. You may find that you have more energy and vitality after completing a detox.

- **Mental Clarity and Focus:** Detoxification can also help to clear mental fog and improve focus and concentration. By removing toxins that cloud the mind, detoxification can enhance your mental clarity and cognitive function.

- **Radiant Skin:** Detoxification supports the health of the skin by promoting the elimination of toxins through the skin and other detoxification organs. This can lead to clearer, brighter, and more radiant skin.

- **Enhanced Immunity:** Regular detoxification helps to support the immune system by removing toxins that can weaken the body's defenses. A strong immune system is essential for preventing illness and maintaining overall health.

- **Emotional Balance:** Detoxification can help to release emotional toxins that contribute to feelings of stress, anxiety, or depression. By clearing these emotional blockages, detoxification can promote greater emotional balance and well-being.

- **Prevention of Chronic Disease:** Regular detoxification helps to prevent the buildup of toxins that can lead to chronic diseases such as heart disease, diabetes, and autoimmune disorders. By keeping your body clean and balanced, you can reduce your risk of developing these conditions.

By incorporating regular detox practices into your lifestyle, you can support your body's natural detoxification processes and maintain optimal health and well-being.

Introduction to Panchakarma

The Five Main Procedures

Panchakarma is the traditional Ayurvedic detoxification and rejuvenation process, designed to cleanse the body of toxins, restore balance, and promote healing. The term "Panchakarma" translates to "five actions," referring to the five main procedures involved in the process. Each procedure is designed to target specific areas of the body and eliminate toxins through natural channels of elimination.

- **Vamana (Therapeutic Emesis):** Vamana involves inducing therapeutic vomiting to eliminate toxins from the upper gastrointestinal tract, particularly the stomach. This procedure is used to treat Kapha-related imbalances such as congestion, asthma, bronchitis, and chronic sinusitis. Vamana helps to clear excess mucus and phlegm, improve respiratory function, and restore balance to the digestive system.

- **Virechana (Therapeutic Purgation):** Virechana is a cleansing procedure that involves the use of herbal laxatives to eliminate toxins from the lower gastrointestinal tract, particularly the intestines. This procedure is used to treat Pitta-related imbalances such as acid reflux, skin disorders, and inflammatory conditions. Virechana helps to clear excess bile and heat from the body, improve digestion, and promote overall detoxification.

- **Basti (Medicated Enema):** Basti is one of the most important procedures in Panchakarma, involving the administration of medicated enemas to cleanse the colon and eliminate toxins from the lower digestive tract. Basti is used to treat Vata-related imbalances such as constipation, arthritis, and nervous system disorders. Basti helps to nourish and strengthen the colon, improve digestion, and support the elimination of waste and toxins.

- **Nasya (Nasal Administration):** Nasya involves the administration of medicated oils or powders through the nasal passages to cleanse the sinuses, throat, and respiratory system. This procedure is used to treat Kapha-related imbalances such as sinus congestion, allergies, and headaches. Nasya helps to clear excess mucus, improve respiratory function, and promote mental clarity.

- **Raktamokshana (Bloodletting):** Raktamokshana is a therapeutic procedure that involves the removal of small amounts of blood to eliminate toxins from the bloodstream. This procedure is used to treat Pitta-related imbalances such as skin disorders, hypertension, and inflammatory conditions. Raktamokshana helps to purify the blood, reduce inflammation, and restore balance to the body.

Each of these procedures is performed under the supervision of a trained Ayurvedic practitioner and is tailored to the individual's specific dosha constitution and health needs. Panchakarma is typically performed over several days or weeks, depending on the individual's condition and the complexity of the detoxification process.

Preparation and Aftercare

Panchakarma is a powerful and intensive detoxification process that requires careful preparation and aftercare to ensure its effectiveness and safety. Proper preparation and aftercare are essential for supporting the body's natural detoxification processes and promoting long-term health.

- **Preparation:** Before undergoing Panchakarma, it is important to prepare the body and mind for the detoxification process. This may involve following a specific diet, known as the "Panchakarma diet," which consists of light, easily digestible foods such as kitchari (a dish made from rice and mung beans), warm soups, and herbal teas. The Panchakarma diet helps to strengthen the digestive fire, reduce Ama, and prepare the body for the elimination of toxins.

    In addition to dietary preparations, the individual may also be advised to undergo "Snehana" (internal and external oleation) and "Swedana" (therapeutic sweating) before the Panchakarma procedures. Snehana involves the use of medicated oils, both internally and externally, to loosen and mobilize toxins from the tissues. Swedana involves the use of steam or heat to open the channels of elimination and promote the release of toxins.

- **Aftercare:** After completing Panchakarma, it is important to follow specific aftercare guidelines to support the body's recovery and maintain the benefits of the detoxification process. This may include following a post-Panchakarma diet that consists of light, nourishing foods, gradually reintroducing regular foods, and avoiding heavy, processed, or fried foods.

  Aftercare may also involve continued use of specific herbs or supplements to support the detoxification process, as well as practices such as yoga, meditation, and pranayama to promote relaxation and mental clarity. The individual may also be advised to avoid strenuous physical activity, stress, and exposure to environmental toxins during the recovery period.

By following these preparation and aftercare guidelines, you can enhance the effectiveness of Panchakarma and promote long-term health and well-being.

At-Home Detox Practices

Simplified Detox Methods

While Panchakarma is a powerful and comprehensive detoxification process, it is not always practical or accessible for everyone. Fortunately, there are several simplified detox methods that can be practiced at home to support the body's natural detoxification processes and promote overall health.

- **Detox Diet:** One of the simplest and most effective ways to detoxify the body at home is to follow a detox diet. A detox diet typically consists of light, easily digestible foods such as kitchari, steamed vegetables, and herbal teas. Avoid processed foods, refined sugars, caffeine, alcohol, and dairy products, as these can contribute to the buildup of toxins. Focus on fresh, organic, and whole foods that nourish the body and support digestion.

- **Oil Pulling:** Oil pulling is a traditional Ayurvedic practice that involves swishing oil (such as sesame or coconut oil) in the mouth for several minutes to remove toxins and improve oral health. Oil pulling helps to eliminate toxins from the mouth, reduce plaque buildup, and promote healthy gums. It can be practiced daily as part of your morning routine.

- **Herbal Teas:** Drinking herbal teas is a gentle and effective way to support detoxification at home. Herbal teas such as ginger, turmeric, dandelion, and fennel help to stimulate digestion, support liver function, and promote the elimination of toxins. Enjoy a cup of herbal tea in the morning or throughout the day to support your body's natural detoxification processes.

- **Dry Brushing:** Dry brushing is a simple and invigorating practice that involves brushing the skin with a dry, natural-bristle brush. This practice helps to stimulate circulation, exfoliate dead skin cells, and promote lymphatic drainage. Dry brushing can be practiced before your morning shower to support detoxification and improve skin health.

- **Epsom Salt Baths:** Taking a warm bath with Epsom salts is a relaxing and detoxifying practice that helps to draw out toxins, reduce inflammation, and soothe sore muscles. Epsom salts are rich in magnesium, which helps to relax the muscles and support the body's detoxification processes. Add a cup of Epsom salts to your bath and soak for 20-30 minutes to promote relaxation and detoxification.

Supporting Long-Term Health

In addition to practicing at-home detox methods, it is important to adopt a lifestyle that supports long-term health and prevents the buildup of toxins. This involves making mindful choices about your diet, lifestyle, and environment to promote balance and well-being.

- **Balanced Diet:** Eating a balanced and nourishing diet is one of the most important ways to support long-term health and prevent the accumulation of toxins. Focus on fresh, organic, and whole foods that are appropriate for your dosha constitution. Avoid processed foods, refined sugars, and unhealthy fats, as these can contribute to the buildup of toxins in the body.

- **Regular Exercise:** Regular physical activity is essential for maintaining balance and supporting the body's natural detoxification processes. Choose activities that are appropriate for your dosha, such as yoga, walking, swimming, or dancing. Regular exercise helps to stimulate circulation, improve digestion, and promote the elimination of toxins.

- **Mindful Living:** Living mindfully involves making conscious choices about your environment, relationships, and daily activities. Practice mindfulness in all areas of your life, from the foods you eat to the thoughts you think. Cultivate positive relationships, manage stress effectively, and create a living environment that supports your well-being.

- **Seasonal Detox:** In Ayurveda, it is recommended to practice detoxification at the change of each season to clear the body of toxins and prepare it for the new season. This can involve following a seasonal detox diet, incorporating seasonal herbs, and practicing seasonal cleansing techniques such as oil pulling, dry brushing, and herbal baths.

By adopting these practices and making mindful choices, you can support long-term health, prevent the buildup of toxins, and promote overall balance and well-being.

In this chapter, we have explored the importance of detoxification in Ayurveda, the principles and procedures of Panchakarma, and at-home detox practices that can support your body's natural detoxification processes. By incorporating regular detox practices into your lifestyle, you can remove toxins, restore balance, and promote long-term health and vitality.

As we move forward, the next chapter will delve into Ayurvedic treatments and therapies, exploring how they can be integrated into your holistic health routine to enhance well-being and address specific health concerns. These treatments will provide additional tools to support your journey to optimal health and balance.

Chapter 8:
Ayurvedic Treatments and Therapies

Ayurveda offers a wide range of treatments and therapies designed to restore balance, promote healing, and enhance overall well-being. These treatments are based on the principles of balancing the doshas and addressing the root causes of disease rather than merely treating symptoms. Whether you are seeking relief from a specific health issue or looking to maintain optimal health, Ayurvedic treatments provide powerful tools to support your journey. In this chapter, we will explore some of the most common Ayurvedic treatments, discuss how to choose the right therapy for your unique needs, and examine how Ayurvedic therapies can be integrated with modern medicine for a holistic approach to health.

Common Ayurvedic Treatments

Shirodhara, Nasya, and Basti

Ayurveda offers a variety of treatments, each with its specific benefits and applications. Among the most widely recognized and practiced are Shirodhara, Nasya, and Basti. These treatments are designed to address different aspects of physical, mental, and emotional health, making them valuable tools in the Ayurvedic healing arsenal.

- **Shirodhara:** Shirodhara is one of the most soothing and calming Ayurvedic treatments, often used to address mental and emotional imbalances. The term "Shirodhara" comes from the Sanskrit words "shiro" (head) and "dhara" (flow), and the treatment involves the continuous pouring of warm, medicated oil over the forehead, specifically the "third eye" area, which is associated with intuition and the mind.

  Shirodhara is particularly beneficial for calming the nervous system, reducing stress, anxiety, and insomnia, and promoting mental clarity. It is also used to alleviate headaches, migraines, and conditions related to Vata and Pitta imbalances. The gentle, rhythmic flow of oil helps to soothe the mind, balance the doshas, and induce a deep state of relaxation.

  The treatment is typically performed in a quiet, comfortable setting, with the individual lying on their back while the warm oil is slowly poured over the forehead. The session usually lasts between 30 to 60 minutes, and the individual may experience a profound sense of calm and well-being during and after the treatment.

- **Nasya:** Nasya is an Ayurvedic treatment that involves the administration of medicated oils, powders, or herbal extracts through the nasal passages. Nasya is used to cleanse and purify the sinuses, enhance respiratory function, and balance the doshas, particularly Kapha and Vata. The nasal passages are considered a direct route to the brain and the central nervous system, making Nasya an effective therapy for mental clarity, emotional balance, and neurological conditions.

  Nasya is commonly used to treat sinus congestion, allergies, headaches, migraines, and conditions such as insomnia and anxiety. It can also be used to enhance memory, concentration, and overall mental function. The treatment typically begins with a facial massage and steam to open the nasal passages, followed by the application of the medicated oil or powder into each nostril. The individual is then instructed to inhale deeply to allow the substance to penetrate the nasal passages and reach the desired areas.

  Regular practice of Nasya can help to prevent respiratory and sinus issues, improve mental clarity, and promote emotional balance. It is a simple yet powerful therapy that can be easily integrated into a daily routine.

- **Basti:** Basti is one of the most important and effective treatments in Ayurveda, often referred to as the "mother of all treatments." It involves the administration of medicated enemas to cleanse and nourish the colon, which is considered the seat of Vata dosha. Basti is used to treat a wide range of conditions related to Vata imbalances, including constipation, arthritis, neurological disorders, and chronic pain.

There are two main types of Basti: "Niruha Basti," which involves the use of a decoction of herbs, and "Anuvasana Basti," which involves the use of medicated oils. Niruha Basti is primarily used for cleansing and detoxification, while Anuvasana Basti is used for nourishment and rejuvenation.

Basti works by balancing Vata dosha, which governs movement and communication in the body. By cleansing the colon and restoring balance to Vata, Basti helps to improve digestion, enhance nutrient absorption, and promote overall health. The treatment is typically administered over a series of sessions, with the specific protocol tailored to the individual's needs.

Benefits and Applications

Each of these Ayurvedic treatments offers unique benefits and applications, making them valuable tools for addressing a wide range of health concerns. Here is a summary of the key benefits and applications of Shirodhara, Nasya, and Basti:

- **Shirodhara:**
    - Benefits: Reduces stress and anxiety, promotes relaxation, improves mental clarity, alleviates headaches and migraines, supports sleep.
    - Applications: Mental and emotional imbalances, insomnia, headaches, Vata and Pitta imbalances.
- **Nasya:**
    - Benefits: Clears sinus congestion, enhances respiratory function, improves mental clarity,

            balances Kapha and Vata, supports neurological health.
        - Applications: Sinus issues, allergies, headaches, respiratory conditions, mental fog, insomnia.
- **Basti:**
    - Benefits: Cleanses the colon, balances Vata dosha, improves digestion, relieves constipation, supports joint and nervous system health.
    - Applications: Vata imbalances, constipation, arthritis, neurological disorders, chronic pain.

These treatments can be used individually or in combination, depending on the individual's needs and the specific dosha imbalances being addressed. When performed under the guidance of a trained Ayurvedic practitioner, these therapies can have profound and lasting effects on overall health and well-being.

Choosing the Right Therapy

Matching Treatments to Dosha Imbalances

One of the key principles of Ayurveda is that treatments and therapies should be tailored to the individual's unique constitution, or "Prakriti," as well as their current state of dosha imbalance, or "Vikriti." Understanding your dominant dosha and any imbalances is essential for choosing the right Ayurvedic treatment to restore balance and promote healing.

- **Vata Imbalances:** Vata imbalances are characterized by dryness, coldness, and irregularity. Common symptoms of Vata imbalance include anxiety, insomnia, constipation, dry skin, and joint pain. Treatments that are grounding, warming, and nourishing are typically recommended for Vata imbalances. Basti, Shirodhara, and Abhyanga (oil massage) are particularly effective for calming Vata and restoring balance.

- **Pitta Imbalances:** Pitta imbalances are characterized by heat, intensity, and inflammation. Common symptoms of Pitta imbalance include acid reflux, skin rashes, irritability, and inflammatory conditions. Treatments that are cooling, soothing, and calming are typically recommended for Pitta imbalances. Shirodhara, Nasya, and cooling herbal therapies are effective for reducing Pitta and promoting harmony.

- **Kapha Imbalances:** Kapha imbalances are characterized by heaviness, stagnation, and congestion. Common symptoms of Kapha imbalance include lethargy, weight gain, sinus congestion, and sluggish digestion. Treatments that are invigorating, stimulating, and cleansing are typically recommended for Kapha imbalances. Nasya, dry brushing, and Udvartana (herbal powder massage) are effective for balancing Kapha and increasing energy.

When choosing an Ayurvedic treatment, it is important to consider both your Prakriti and Vikriti. An Ayurvedic practitioner can help assess your dosha constitution and recommend the most appropriate therapies to address your specific needs. In some cases, a combination of treatments may be recommended to achieve the best results.

Professional vs. At-Home Therapies

While many Ayurvedic treatments are best performed by trained professionals, there are also several therapies that can be safely and effectively practiced at home. Understanding the difference between professional and at-home therapies can help you make informed decisions about your health and well-being.

- **Professional Therapies:** Professional Ayurvedic treatments, such as Panchakarma, Shirodhara, and Basti, are typically performed in a clinical or spa setting by trained Ayurvedic practitioners. These treatments often involve specialized equipment, medicated oils, and precise techniques that require professional expertise. Professional therapies are recommended for individuals with specific health concerns, severe dosha imbalances, or those seeking a comprehensive detoxification and rejuvenation program.

  The benefits of professional therapies include personalized care, access to high-quality Ayurvedic products, and the expertise of a trained practitioner who can tailor the treatment to your unique needs. Professional treatments are often more intensive and can provide deeper and longer-lasting effects.

- **At-Home Therapies:** At-home Ayurvedic therapies are more accessible and can be easily integrated into your daily routine. These therapies may include practices such as Abhyanga (self-massage), Nasya (nasal administration), oil pulling, and herbal teas. While at-home therapies may not be as intensive as professional treatments, they offer the advantage of being more convenient and cost-effective.

  At-home therapies are particularly beneficial for maintaining balance between professional treatments, supporting daily detoxification, and promoting overall health. They are also a great way to incorporate Ayurvedic principles into your everyday life and take a proactive approach to your well-being.

When deciding between professional and at-home therapies, consider your specific health needs, goals, and lifestyle. For more serious or complex health concerns, professional treatments may be necessary, while at-home therapies can be an excellent way to support your health on a daily basis.

Integrating Ayurvedic and Modern Therapies

Complementary Approaches

Ayurveda and modern medicine can work together as complementary approaches to health and healing. While Ayurveda focuses on restoring balance and preventing disease through holistic practices, modern medicine excels in diagnosing and treating acute and severe conditions. By integrating these two approaches, you can create a comprehensive and personalized healthcare plan that addresses both the root causes of illness and the symptoms.

- **Chronic Conditions:** For chronic conditions such as diabetes, arthritis, or digestive disorders, Ayurveda can offer supportive therapies that complement conventional medical treatments. For example, Ayurvedic dietary recommendations, herbal supplements, and detoxification therapies can help to manage symptoms, reduce inflammation, and improve overall quality of life. These therapies can be used alongside prescribed medications to enhance their effectiveness and minimize side effects.

- **Stress and Mental Health:** Ayurveda offers powerful tools for managing stress and promoting mental health, including meditation, yoga, and herbal therapies. These practices can be integrated with modern therapeutic approaches such as cognitive-behavioral therapy (CBT) or pharmacotherapy to provide a more holistic approach to mental health care. Ayurvedic therapies can help to address the underlying imbalances that contribute to stress and mental health issues, supporting long-term recovery and well-being.

- **Post-Surgery Recovery:** After surgery, Ayurveda can play a valuable role in supporting recovery and promoting healing. Ayurvedic treatments such as Abhyanga, herbal supplements, and gentle yoga can help to reduce inflammation, improve circulation, and restore strength and vitality. These therapies can complement conventional post-surgery care, helping to speed up recovery and reduce the risk of complications.

By integrating Ayurvedic and modern therapies, you can create a balanced and comprehensive approach to health that addresses both the physical and emotional aspects of well-being.

Case Studies and Success Stories

The integration of Ayurvedic and modern therapies has led to numerous success stories, demonstrating the power of a holistic approach to health. Here are a few examples:

- **Case Study 1: Chronic Digestive Issues**
  - A 45-year-old woman with chronic irritable bowel syndrome (IBS) sought Ayurvedic treatment after experiencing limited relief from conventional medications. After undergoing a comprehensive Panchakarma detoxification program, combined with dietary changes and herbal supplements, the patient reported significant improvements in her digestion, reduced bloating and discomfort, and improved energy levels. By continuing to follow Ayurvedic dietary recommendations and incorporating regular detox practices, the patient was able to maintain her digestive health and reduce her reliance on medication.

- **Case Study 2: Stress and Anxiety**
  - A 32-year-old man with a history of anxiety and panic attacks sought Ayurvedic treatment alongside his conventional therapy. Through the use of Shirodhara, regular meditation, and adaptogenic herbs such as Ashwagandha, the patient experienced a marked reduction in anxiety symptoms, improved sleep quality, and increased resilience to stress. The combination of Ayurvedic therapies and cognitive-behavioral therapy (CBT) provided a comprehensive approach to managing his anxiety, leading to lasting improvements in his mental health.

- **Case Study 3: Post-Surgery Recovery**
  - A 60-year-old man recovering from knee replacement surgery sought Ayurvedic support to aid in his recovery. With the guidance of an

Ayurvedic practitioner, the patient incorporated Abhyanga (oil massage), herbal supplements, and gentle yoga into his post-surgery care. These therapies helped to reduce inflammation, improve circulation, and restore mobility, leading to a faster and more comfortable recovery. The patient reported improved joint function, reduced pain, and a greater sense of overall well-being.

These case studies highlight the potential of integrating Ayurvedic and modern therapies to achieve optimal health outcomes. By addressing both the root causes of illness and the symptoms, this holistic approach provides a more comprehensive and effective path to healing.

In this chapter, we have explored the range of Ayurvedic treatments and therapies available to support your health and well-being. We discussed common Ayurvedic treatments such as Shirodhara, Nasya, and Basti, and provided guidance on choosing the right therapy based on your dosha imbalances and specific health needs. We also examined how Ayurvedic and modern therapies can be integrated to create a complementary approach to health, supported by real-life case studies and success stories.

As we move forward, the next chapter will delve into emotional and mental health in Ayurveda, exploring how Ayurvedic practices can support mental clarity, emotional balance, and overall well-being. By understanding the mind-body connection and the role of the doshas in mental health, you can create a holistic approach to emotional wellness.

Chapter 9: Emotional and Mental Health in Ayurveda

Ayurveda, with its holistic approach to health, recognizes the profound connection between the mind, body, and spirit. Emotional and mental health are seen as integral to overall well-being, and maintaining balance in these areas is essential for a fulfilling and harmonious life. In this chapter, we will explore the Ayurvedic view on mental health, focusing on the mind-body connection and the importance of emotional balance. We will also discuss Ayurvedic strategies for managing stress and anxiety, and provide guidance on enhancing mental clarity and focus through practices, nutrition, and herbal support.

Ayurvedic View on Mental Health

Understanding the Mind-Body Connection

In Ayurveda, the mind and body are viewed as deeply interconnected, with each influencing the health and functioning of the other. The concept of "Sattva," "Rajas," and "Tamas" is central to understanding the mind in Ayurveda. These three qualities, or "Gunas," govern the mental and emotional state of an individual:

- **Sattva (Purity and Harmony):** Sattva represents clarity, purity, and balance. A Sattvic mind is calm, focused, and full of wisdom and compassion. Sattva is associated with mental clarity, emotional stability, and a deep sense of inner peace. Cultivating Sattva is considered essential for maintaining mental and emotional health.

- **Rajas (Activity and Passion):** Rajas is the quality of activity, movement, and restlessness. A Rajasic mind is driven by desire, ambition, and a constant need for stimulation. While Rajas can lead to creativity and achievement, it can also result in stress, anxiety, and emotional instability when out of balance. Excessive Rajas can cause the mind to become agitated and overactive, leading to mental and emotional disturbances.

- **Tamas (Inertia and Ignorance):** Tamas represents darkness, inertia, and ignorance. A Tamasic mind is dull, lethargic, and prone to confusion and negativity. When Tamas dominates, it can lead to depression, apathy, and a lack of motivation. Excessive Tamas can cloud the mind, making it difficult to think clearly or take positive action.

The goal in Ayurveda is to cultivate Sattva while balancing Rajas and Tamas. By fostering a Sattvic mind, you can achieve mental clarity, emotional stability, and a sense of inner peace. This balance is essential for overall well-being and is achieved through a combination of diet, lifestyle practices, meditation, and mindfulness.

Importance of Emotional Balance

Emotional balance is a key component of mental health in Ayurveda. Emotions are seen as a natural part of the human experience, but when they become overwhelming or imbalanced, they can lead to physical and mental health issues. Ayurveda teaches that emotions should be acknowledged and processed in a healthy way, rather than suppressed or allowed to spiral out of control.

Each dosha has a tendency toward certain emotional patterns:

- **Vata:** When in balance, Vata types are creative, enthusiastic, and adaptable. However, when out of balance, they can become anxious, fearful, and scattered. Vata imbalances often manifest as restlessness, insomnia, and feelings of insecurity.

- **Pitta:** Balanced Pitta individuals are focused, determined, and confident. When imbalanced, they may become irritable, angry, and overly critical. Pitta imbalances can lead to stress, frustration, and a tendency toward perfectionism.

- **Kapha:** When balanced, Kapha types are calm, compassionate, and nurturing. However, when out of balance, they can become lethargic, resistant to change, and prone to depression. Kapha imbalances often result in feelings of heaviness, stagnation, and attachment.

Maintaining emotional balance involves understanding your dominant dosha and its tendencies, and using Ayurvedic practices to keep your emotions in check. This may include dietary adjustments, lifestyle changes, meditation, and the use of specific herbs to support emotional well-being.

Managing Stress and Anxiety

Ayurvedic Strategies for Stress Relief

Stress and anxiety are common issues in modern life, but Ayurveda offers a range of strategies to help manage these challenges and restore balance. By addressing the root causes of stress and anxiety, Ayurveda provides tools to calm the mind, soothe the nervous system, and promote a sense of peace and relaxation.

- **Meditation and Mindfulness:** Meditation is one of the most effective ways to manage stress and anxiety in Ayurveda. Regular meditation helps to calm the mind, reduce mental chatter, and cultivate a sense of inner peace. Mindfulness practices, which involve bringing full awareness to the present moment, can also help to reduce stress by breaking the cycle of negative thinking and promoting a sense of calm and clarity.

- **Pranayama (Breathing Exercises):** Pranayama, or breath control, is another powerful tool for managing stress and anxiety. Techniques such as Nadi Shodhana (alternate nostril breathing) and Bhramari (bee breath) help to calm the nervous system, balance the doshas, and reduce mental agitation. Regular practice of Pranayama can enhance emotional resilience and promote a sense of well-being.

- **Abhyanga (Self-Massage):** Abhyanga, or self-massage with warm oil, is a deeply soothing practice that helps to calm the nervous system and reduce stress. The application of warm oil to the skin nourishes the tissues, enhances circulation, and promotes relaxation. Abhyanga is particularly beneficial for calming Vata dosha, which is often associated with anxiety and restlessness.

- **Yoga:** Yoga is a holistic practice that combines physical postures, breathwork, and meditation to promote mental and emotional balance. Specific yoga poses can help to release tension, calm the mind, and restore balance to the doshas. For example, forward bends and restorative poses are particularly effective for calming the nervous system and reducing stress.

- **Herbal Support:** Ayurveda offers a variety of herbs that can help to manage stress and anxiety. Adaptogenic herbs such as Ashwagandha, Brahmi, and Jatamansi are particularly effective for calming the mind, reducing stress, and promoting emotional balance. These herbs can be taken in the form of teas, capsules, or tinctures, and are often used in combination with other Ayurvedic practices.

Herbs and Lifestyle Modifications

In addition to the strategies mentioned above, specific herbs and lifestyle modifications can play a crucial role in managing stress and anxiety in Ayurveda. By incorporating these practices into your daily routine, you can create a more balanced and peaceful life.

- **Ashwagandha:** Ashwagandha is one of the most revered adaptogenic herbs in Ayurveda, known for its ability to reduce stress, anxiety, and fatigue. It helps to balance Vata and Kapha doshas and supports the body's natural response to stress. Ashwagandha can be taken as a supplement, in the form of a powder, capsule, or tincture.

- **Brahmi:** Brahmi is another powerful herb for managing stress and anxiety, particularly in Pitta and Vata types. It is known for its calming and rejuvenating properties, and it helps to enhance mental clarity, focus, and memory. Brahmi can be consumed as a tea, capsule, or in a traditional Ayurvedic formulation such as Brahmi Ghrita (medicated ghee).

- **Jatamansi:** Jatamansi is a calming herb that is particularly effective for reducing anxiety, promoting restful sleep, and balancing the nervous system. It is especially beneficial for Vata and Pitta imbalances and can be used in the form of a tincture, powder, or essential oil.

- **Dietary Adjustments:** Your diet plays a crucial role in managing stress and anxiety in Ayurveda. Eating a balanced, nourishing diet that is appropriate for your dosha can help to calm the mind and support emotional balance. For example, Vata types benefit from warm, grounding foods, while Pitta types should focus on cooling, soothing foods. Kapha types can benefit from light, invigorating foods that promote energy and vitality.

- **Routine and Structure:** Establishing a regular daily routine, or Dinacharya, is essential for managing stress and anxiety. A consistent routine helps to ground the mind, reduce mental agitation, and promote a sense of stability. This may include regular meal times, a consistent sleep schedule, and daily practices such as meditation, yoga, and self-care.

By combining these herbs and lifestyle modifications with other Ayurvedic practices, you can effectively manage stress and anxiety and create a more balanced and harmonious life.

Enhancing Mental Clarity and Focus

Practices for Mental Agility

Mental clarity and focus are essential for navigating the complexities of modern life. Ayurveda offers a range of practices to enhance mental agility, sharpen concentration, and promote cognitive function. By incorporating these practices into your daily routine, you can improve your mental performance and maintain a clear, focused mind.

- **Meditation:** Regular meditation is one of the most effective ways to enhance mental clarity and focus. By calming the mind and reducing distractions, meditation helps to improve concentration and cognitive function. Techniques such as mindfulness meditation, mantra meditation, and focused attention meditation are particularly beneficial for sharpening the mind and enhancing mental agility.

- **Pranayama:** Breath control practices, or Pranayama, are powerful tools for enhancing mental clarity and focus. Techniques such as Kapalabhati (skull-shining breath) and Bhastrika (bellows breath) help to energize the mind, increase oxygen flow to the brain, and improve mental performance. Regular practice of Pranayama can also help to reduce mental fatigue and enhance cognitive function.

- **Trataka (Candle Gazing):** Trataka is a traditional Ayurvedic practice that involves gazing at a fixed point, such as a candle flame, to improve concentration and mental clarity. This practice helps to calm the mind, enhance focus, and sharpen visual perception. Trataka can be practiced for a few minutes each day as part of your meditation routine.

- **Yoga:** Specific yoga poses can help to enhance mental clarity and focus by increasing blood flow to the brain and calming the nervous system. Inversions such as Shoulder Stand (Sarvangasana) and Headstand (Sirsasana), as well as poses like Tree Pose (Vrksasana) and Warrior III (Virabhadrasana III), are particularly effective for improving concentration and cognitive function.

Nutrition and Herbal Support

In addition to practices that enhance mental clarity and focus, Ayurveda emphasizes the importance of proper nutrition and herbal support. A diet that nourishes the mind and body, combined with the use of specific herbs, can help to enhance cognitive function and promote mental agility.

- **Sattvic Diet:** A Sattvic diet is recommended in Ayurveda for promoting mental clarity, focus, and spiritual growth. This diet emphasizes fresh, organic, and plant-based foods that are easy to digest and free from toxins. Sattvic foods include fruits, vegetables, whole grains, nuts, seeds, and dairy products such as ghee and milk. Avoiding stimulants such as caffeine, alcohol, and processed foods is also important for maintaining mental clarity.

- **Brahmi:** Brahmi is one of the most important herbs in Ayurveda for enhancing mental clarity and cognitive function. It is known for its ability to improve memory, concentration, and mental agility. Brahmi can be consumed in the form of a tea, capsule, or in traditional Ayurvedic formulations such as Brahmi Ghrita.

- **Gotu Kola:** Gotu Kola is another powerful herb for enhancing cognitive function and mental clarity. It is known for its ability to improve memory, focus, and mental agility. Gotu Kola is particularly beneficial for balancing Pitta and Kapha doshas and can be taken as a supplement, in the form of a powder, capsule, or tincture.

- **Shankhapushpi:** Shankhapushpi is a traditional Ayurvedic herb that is used to enhance memory, concentration, and cognitive function. It is particularly effective for balancing Vata and Pitta doshas and is often used in combination with other herbs such as Brahmi and Gotu Kola. Shankhapushpi can be taken as a tea, capsule, or in traditional Ayurvedic formulations.

- **Nuts and Seeds:** Nuts and seeds are rich in essential fatty acids, which are important for brain health and cognitive function. Almonds, walnuts, flaxseeds, and chia seeds are particularly beneficial for enhancing mental clarity and focus. These foods can be incorporated into your diet as snacks, added to smoothies, or used as toppings for salads and other dishes.

By combining these practices, nutrition, and herbal support, you can enhance your mental clarity and focus, improve cognitive function, and maintain a sharp, agile mind.

In this chapter, we have explored the Ayurvedic approach to emotional and mental health, focusing on the mind-body connection, the importance of emotional balance, and strategies for managing stress and anxiety. We also discussed practices, nutrition, and herbal support for enhancing mental clarity and focus. By incorporating these Ayurvedic principles into your daily life, you can create a holistic approach to mental and emotional well-being, supporting both your physical and spiritual health.

As we move forward, we will explore how Ayurvedic practices can support hormonal balance, reproductive health, and overall vitality throughout the different stages of a woman's life. By understanding the unique needs of women's health, you can apply Ayurvedic wisdom to promote balance, strength, and well-being at every age.

Chapter 10: Women's Health and Ayurveda

Women's health in Ayurveda is approached with a deep understanding of the unique physiological and emotional needs that women experience throughout their lives. Ayurveda emphasizes the importance of maintaining balance, particularly with respect to hormonal health, reproductive well-being, and the various stages of a woman's life, including menstruation, pregnancy, and menopause. This chapter will explore the specific needs of women's health, offer Ayurvedic practices tailored to women, and provide guidance on pregnancy and postpartum care. By integrating these Ayurvedic principles into daily life, women can achieve greater balance, vitality, and overall well-being.

Unique Needs of Women's Health

Hormonal Balance and Reproductive Health

Hormonal balance is central to women's health and well-being. In Ayurveda, hormones are governed by the doshas, particularly Pitta, which is responsible for metabolic and transformative processes in the body. When the doshas are balanced, hormones function harmoniously, supporting everything from mood and energy levels to reproductive health.

- **Pitta and Hormonal Health:** Pitta governs the endocrine system, which includes the production and regulation of hormones. An imbalance in Pitta can lead to issues such as hot flashes, irritability, inflammation, and conditions like polycystic ovary syndrome (PCOS) and thyroid disorders. Balancing Pitta through cooling, calming practices and diet is essential for maintaining hormonal health.

- **Vata and Menstrual Health:** Vata is responsible for movement in the body, including the flow of the menstrual cycle. An imbalanced Vata can lead to irregular or painful periods, anxiety, and dryness. Nourishing, grounding, and warming practices can help to balance Vata and support regular, healthy menstrual cycles.

- **Kapha and Reproductive Health:** Kapha governs the structure and stability of the body, including the reproductive tissues. When Kapha is in balance, it supports fertility, strong reproductive tissues, and healthy pregnancies. However, excess Kapha can lead to stagnation, weight gain, and conditions such as cysts or fibroids. Stimulating and invigorating practices are key to balancing Kapha and supporting reproductive health.

Menstrual Health and Menopause

Ayurveda places significant importance on menstrual health as a reflection of a woman's overall well-being. The menstrual cycle, known as "Artava," is considered a natural detoxification process that supports the balance of the doshas and the health of the reproductive system.

- **Menstrual Health:** A regular, pain-free menstrual cycle is a sign of balanced doshas and good health. However, imbalances in Vata, Pitta, or Kapha can lead to menstrual irregularities such as dysmenorrhea (painful periods), amenorrhea (absence of periods), or menorrhagia (heavy bleeding). Ayurveda recommends specific dietary, lifestyle, and herbal practices to support menstrual health. For example, warm, nourishing foods and gentle exercise can help balance Vata during menstruation, while cooling and hydrating foods can help manage Pitta-related symptoms such as inflammation or irritability.

- **Menopause:** Menopause, or the transition out of the reproductive years, is seen in Ayurveda as a natural and important stage of a woman's life. This transition is often governed by Vata dosha, leading to symptoms such as hot flashes, mood swings, and dryness. Ayurveda offers a holistic approach to menopause, emphasizing the importance of balancing Vata through diet, lifestyle practices, and herbal support. For example, incorporating warm, oily, and grounding foods can help soothe Vata, while herbs such as Shatavari and Ashwagandha can support hormonal balance and overall well-being during this transition.

Ayurvedic Practices for Women

Tailored Nutrition and Lifestyle

Ayurveda emphasizes the importance of tailored nutrition and lifestyle practices to support women's unique health needs. By understanding your dosha constitution and any current imbalances, you can create a diet and lifestyle plan that promotes hormonal balance, reproductive health, and overall well-being.

- **Nutrition:** A balanced diet that is appropriate for your dosha is essential for supporting women's health. Vata types benefit from warm, nourishing foods such as cooked grains, soups, and stews, while Pitta types should focus on cooling, hydrating foods like fresh fruits, vegetables, and leafy greens. Kapha types can benefit from light, spicy, and invigorating foods that promote digestion and metabolism. Specific foods such as sesame seeds, almonds, and leafy greens are particularly beneficial for supporting hormonal health and reproductive function.

- **Lifestyle:** Lifestyle practices are also key to maintaining women's health. Regular physical activity, such as yoga or walking, is important for balancing the doshas and supporting overall vitality. Vata types should focus on gentle, grounding exercises, while Pitta types can benefit from moderate, cooling activities. Kapha types may need more vigorous, stimulating exercises to boost energy and metabolism. Additionally, maintaining a regular sleep schedule, practicing stress management techniques such as meditation or pranayama, and creating a supportive daily routine (Dinacharya) are all important for promoting women's health.

Herbal Support and Therapies

Ayurveda offers a wide range of herbal support and therapies specifically tailored to women's health. These herbs can help to balance hormones, support reproductive health, and manage symptoms related to menstruation, menopause, and other stages of life.

- **Shatavari:** Shatavari is one of the most revered herbs in Ayurveda for women's health. It is known as a powerful adaptogen that supports hormonal balance, reproductive health, and overall vitality. Shatavari is particularly beneficial for balancing Pitta and Vata doshas and can be used to manage menstrual irregularities, menopausal symptoms, and issues related to fertility. It is often taken in the form of a powder, capsule, or herbal tea.

- **Ashwagandha:** Ashwagandha is another important herb for women's health, known for its ability to reduce stress, support the nervous system, and promote hormonal balance. It is particularly beneficial for managing symptoms of menopause, such as hot flashes and mood swings, and for supporting overall energy levels and vitality. Ashwagandha can be taken as a supplement, in the form of a powder, capsule, or tincture.

- **Guggulu:** Guggulu is an Ayurvedic herb commonly used to support metabolism, detoxification, and reproductive health. It is particularly beneficial for balancing Kapha dosha and can be used to manage conditions such as PCOS, fibroids, and weight gain. Guggulu can be taken as a supplement, in the form of a powder, capsule, or as part of a traditional Ayurvedic formulation.

- **Chyawanprash:** Chyawanprash is a traditional Ayurvedic herbal jam that is particularly beneficial for women's health. It is rich in antioxidants, vitamins, and minerals and supports overall vitality, immunity, and reproductive health. Chyawanprash can be taken daily as a supplement to support energy levels, hormonal balance, and overall well-being.

In addition to these herbs, specific Ayurvedic therapies such as Abhyanga (self-massage with warm oil), Shirodhara (oil therapy for the head), and Bastis (medicated enemas) can be used to support women's health. These therapies help to balance the doshas, promote relaxation, and support reproductive health.

Pregnancy and Postpartum Care

Ayurvedic Prenatal Practices

Pregnancy is a sacred time in a woman's life, and Ayurveda offers a range of practices to support both the mother and the developing baby. The focus during pregnancy is on nurturing the body and mind, maintaining balance, and preparing for a healthy and smooth delivery.

- **Nourishing Diet:** During pregnancy, it is essential to follow a nourishing diet that supports both the mother and the growing baby. Ayurveda recommends warm, cooked foods that are easy to digest and rich in nutrients. Foods such as ghee, milk, almonds, dates, and leafy greens are particularly beneficial. Hydration is also important, and the mother should drink plenty of water, herbal teas, and warm milk.

- **Gentle Exercise:** Regular gentle exercise, such as prenatal yoga or walking, is recommended during pregnancy to promote circulation, reduce stress, and prepare the body for childbirth. Vata types should focus on grounding exercises, while Pitta types can benefit from cooling, moderate activities. Kapha types may need more stimulating exercises to boost energy levels and maintain a healthy weight.

- **Herbal Support:** Ayurveda recommends specific herbs to support pregnancy, such as Shatavari, which nourishes the reproductive tissues and supports hormonal balance, and Bala, which strengthens the body and supports the developing baby. These herbs can be taken as part of a prenatal regimen, in consultation with an Ayurvedic practitioner.

- **Relaxation and Stress Management:** Managing stress during pregnancy is crucial for the health of both the mother and the baby. Practices such as meditation, deep breathing exercises, and self-massage with warm oil (Abhyanga) can help to reduce stress, promote relaxation, and prepare the mind and body for childbirth.

Postnatal Recovery and Wellness

The postpartum period, known as "Sutika Kala" in Ayurveda, is a time of significant transformation and recovery for the new mother. Ayurvedic postpartum care focuses on nourishing and rejuvenating the mother's body, supporting breastfeeding, and promoting emotional well-being.

- **Nourishing Diet:** After childbirth, it is essential to follow a nourishing diet that supports the mother's recovery and promotes lactation. Ayurveda recommends warm, easily digestible foods such as kitchari (a dish made from rice and mung beans), soups, and stews. Ghee, milk, and herbal teas are also important for nourishing the body and supporting digestion. Spices such as turmeric, ginger, and fennel can be added to the diet to support healing and lactation.

- **Herbal Support:** Specific Ayurvedic herbs can help to support postpartum recovery and wellness. Shatavari is particularly beneficial for promoting lactation and balancing hormones, while Ashwagandha helps to reduce stress and support energy levels. Bala can be used to strengthen the body and promote overall vitality. These herbs can be taken as part of a postpartum regimen, in consultation with an Ayurvedic practitioner.

- **Abhyanga (Self-Massage):** Regular self-massage with warm oil (Abhyanga) is highly recommended during the postpartum period. Abhyanga helps to nourish the body, reduce stress, and promote relaxation. It is particularly beneficial for balancing Vata dosha, which can be elevated after childbirth.

- **Rest and Relaxation:** Rest is crucial during the postpartum period, and Ayurveda emphasizes the importance of giving the body time to heal and rejuvenate. New mothers should prioritize rest, avoid strenuous activities, and create a supportive environment that allows for relaxation and bonding with the baby.

- **Emotional Support:** The postpartum period can be emotionally challenging, and Ayurveda recognizes the importance of emotional support for new mothers. Practices such as meditation, deep breathing exercises, and spending time in nature can help to promote emotional balance and well-being. Support from family, friends, and healthcare professionals is also essential for a smooth and healthy postpartum recovery.

By following these Ayurvedic practices during pregnancy and postpartum, women can support their health and well-being, promote a healthy pregnancy and childbirth, and ensure a smooth and rejuvenating recovery.

In this chapter, we have explored the unique needs of women's health in Ayurveda, focusing on hormonal balance, reproductive health, menstrual health, and menopause. We also discussed tailored Ayurvedic practices for women, including nutrition, lifestyle, herbal support, and therapies. Finally, we provided guidance on Ayurvedic prenatal and postpartum care to support a healthy pregnancy, childbirth, and recovery.

As we move forward, we will explore how Ayurvedic practices can address the specific health needs of men, focusing on energy, vitality, and maintaining balance throughout different stages of life. By understanding and applying these principles, you can support overall well-being and long-term health.

Chapter 11:
Men's Health and Ayurveda

Men's health in Ayurveda is approached with a focus on maintaining energy, vitality, and balance throughout life. Ayurveda recognizes that men have unique health needs, particularly in areas such as hormonal balance, reproductive health, and physical strength. By understanding these needs and integrating Ayurvedic practices into daily life, men can achieve optimal health and well-being. In this chapter, we will explore the specific health needs of men, discuss Ayurvedic strategies for maintaining vitality and balance, and provide guidance on promoting longevity and lifelong health. Through these practices, men can cultivate a strong, healthy body and mind, and enjoy a fulfilling and active life.

Focus on Men's Health Needs

Energy and Vitality

Energy and vitality are central to men's health in Ayurveda. The ability to maintain physical strength, mental clarity, and sexual vitality throughout life is considered a key aspect of overall well-being. Ayurveda offers specific practices and recommendations to support these areas, focusing on the balance of the doshas, proper nutrition, and lifestyle habits.

- **Vata and Energy Levels:** Vata dosha governs movement and energy in the body. When Vata is balanced, men experience steady energy levels, creativity, and mental agility. However, when Vata is imbalanced, it can lead to fatigue, restlessness, and difficulty concentrating. To maintain energy levels, it is important to balance Vata through grounding practices, nourishing foods, and regular routines.

- **Pitta and Vitality:** Pitta dosha is responsible for metabolism and transformation in the body. A balanced Pitta supports strong digestion, a healthy metabolism, and vibrant energy. However, an excess of Pitta can lead to burnout, irritability, and inflammation. Cooling and calming practices, along with a balanced diet, are essential for maintaining Pitta and supporting vitality.

- **Kapha and Physical Strength:** Kapha dosha governs structure, stability, and strength in the body. When Kapha is balanced, men experience physical endurance, strong immunity, and emotional stability. However, an excess of Kapha can lead to sluggishness, weight gain, and lethargy. Stimulating and invigorating practices are key to balancing Kapha and maintaining physical strength and vitality.

Reproductive Health and Hormonal Balance

Reproductive health and hormonal balance are critical components of men's health in Ayurveda. The health of the reproductive system is linked to overall vitality and well-being, and maintaining balance in this area is essential for long-term health.

- **Shukra Dhatu (Reproductive Tissue):** In Ayurveda, Shukra Dhatu refers to the reproductive tissue that is responsible for sperm production and sexual vitality. Maintaining the health of Shukra Dhatu is essential for reproductive health and overall vitality. Ayurveda emphasizes the importance of nourishing Shukra Dhatu through proper diet, lifestyle practices, and herbal support.

- **Hormonal Balance:** Hormonal balance is essential for men's health, particularly in relation to testosterone levels, which play a key role in energy, muscle mass, libido, and mood. Ayurveda offers specific strategies to support hormonal balance, including diet, exercise, and the use of adaptogenic herbs. Balancing the doshas, particularly Pitta, is important for maintaining healthy hormone levels and preventing conditions such as stress-related hormonal imbalances.

- **Sexual Health:** Ayurveda views sexual health as an integral part of overall well-being. Maintaining sexual vitality and function is important for physical and emotional health. Ayurveda offers specific practices and herbs to support sexual health, including those that enhance libido, improve stamina, and promote healthy reproductive function.

Ayurvedic Strategies for Men

Diet and Exercise Recommendations

Ayurveda emphasizes the importance of diet and exercise in maintaining men's health. By tailoring these practices to an individual's dosha constitution, men can support their energy levels, physical strength, and overall well-being.

- **Diet for Men's Health:** A balanced diet that supports the doshas is essential for maintaining energy, vitality, and hormonal balance. Men should focus on nutrient-dense foods that provide sustained energy and support muscle mass and strength.

    - **Vata Types:** Vata types benefit from warm, nourishing foods that are grounding and easy to digest. Cooked grains, root vegetables, nuts, seeds, and healthy fats such as ghee and olive oil are ideal. Avoid cold, raw, and dry foods, which can aggravate Vata.

    - **Pitta Types:** Pitta types should focus on cooling, hydrating foods that soothe the digestive system and reduce inflammation. Fresh fruits, vegetables, leafy greens, and whole grains are beneficial. Avoid spicy, oily, and acidic foods, which can aggravate Pitta.

    - **Kapha Types:** Kapha types benefit from light, spicy, and invigorating foods that boost metabolism and prevent stagnation. Lean proteins, spicy vegetables, legumes, and whole grains are ideal. Avoid heavy, oily, and sweet foods, which can aggravate Kapha.

Additionally, Ayurveda recommends that men consume foods that are rich in essential fatty acids, protein, and antioxidants, such as avocados, almonds, walnuts, and dark leafy greens, to support overall health and vitality.

- **Exercise for Men's Health:** Regular physical activity is essential for maintaining energy, strength, and vitality. Ayurveda recommends that men choose exercises that are appropriate for their dosha constitution and fitness goals.

    - **Vata Types:** Vata types should engage in gentle, grounding exercises such as yoga, walking, and swimming. These activities help to calm the nervous system and maintain flexibility without causing strain or depletion.

    - **Pitta Types:** Pitta types benefit from moderate-intensity exercises such as cycling, running, and swimming. These activities help to release excess heat and energy, promote endurance, and maintain a balanced metabolism.

    - **Kapha Types:** Kapha types should engage in vigorous, stimulating exercises such as weightlifting, aerobics, and high-intensity interval training (HIIT). These activities help to boost metabolism, reduce weight gain, and prevent lethargy.

In addition to regular exercise, Ayurveda recommends incorporating practices such as Pranayama (breath control) and meditation into your routine to enhance mental clarity, reduce stress, and promote overall well-being.

Herbal Support and Treatments

Ayurveda offers a range of herbs and treatments specifically tailored to support men's health. These herbs help to balance the doshas, support hormonal health, and promote energy, vitality, and reproductive health.

- **Ashwagandha:** Ashwagandha is one of the most important herbs in Ayurveda for men's health. It is known for its adaptogenic properties, which help to reduce stress, enhance stamina, and support hormonal balance. Ashwagandha is particularly beneficial for boosting energy levels, improving muscle mass, and enhancing sexual vitality. It can be taken in the form of a powder, capsule, or tincture.

- **Shilajit:** Shilajit is a powerful Ayurvedic tonic known for its rejuvenating and revitalizing properties. It is particularly beneficial for enhancing energy, stamina, and sexual health. Shilajit supports the production of testosterone, improves fertility, and promotes overall vitality. It is often taken as a supplement in the form of a resin, powder, or capsule.

- **Tribulus (Gokshura):** Tribulus, also known as Gokshura, is an Ayurvedic herb that supports male reproductive health and vitality. It is known for its ability to enhance libido, improve sperm quality, and support hormonal balance. Tribulus is particularly beneficial for balancing Pitta and Kapha doshas and can be taken as a supplement in the form of a powder, capsule, or tincture.

- **Kapikacchu (Mucuna Pruriens):** Kapikacchu, also known as Mucuna Pruriens, is an Ayurvedic herb that supports male reproductive health and vitality. It is known for its ability to enhance libido, improve sperm quality, and support healthy testosterone levels. Kapikacchu is particularly beneficial for balancing Vata and Pitta doshas and can be taken as a supplement in the form of a powder, capsule, or tincture.

- **Abhyanga (Self-Massage):** Regular self-massage with warm oil (Abhyanga) is highly recommended for men's health. Abhyanga helps to nourish the tissues, improve circulation, and promote relaxation. It is particularly beneficial for balancing Vata dosha and supporting physical strength and vitality.

In addition to these herbs and treatments, specific Ayurvedic therapies such as Shirodhara (oil therapy for the head), Basti (medicated enemas), and Rasayana (rejuvenation therapies) can be used to support men's health. These therapies help to balance the doshas, promote relaxation, and support overall vitality.

Promoting Longevity and Vitality

Practices for Lifelong Health

Ayurveda emphasizes the importance of maintaining balance and vitality throughout life. By incorporating specific practices into your daily routine, you can promote lifelong health, prevent disease, and enjoy a fulfilling and active life.

- **Dinacharya (Daily Routine):** Establishing a regular daily routine, or Dinacharya, is essential for maintaining balance and vitality. This routine should include regular meal times, physical activity, and self-care practices such as Abhyanga (self-massage) and meditation. A consistent routine helps to ground the mind, reduce stress, and promote overall well-being.

- **Seasonal Adjustments:** Ayurveda recommends adjusting your diet and lifestyle according to the seasons to maintain balance and vitality. For example, during the winter, it is important to focus on warm, nourishing foods and grounding practices to balance Vata dosha. In the summer, cooling and hydrating foods and activities help to balance Pitta dosha. In the spring, light, invigorating foods and practices support the detoxification and balance of Kapha dosha.

- **Stress Management:** Managing stress is essential for maintaining vitality and preventing disease. Regular practice of meditation, Pranayama (breath control), and yoga can help to reduce stress, calm the mind, and promote emotional balance. Adaptogenic herbs such as Ashwagandha and Brahmi can also support the body's natural response to stress.

- **Rejuvenation Therapies (Rasayana):** Rasayana therapies are an important aspect of Ayurvedic practice for promoting longevity and vitality. These therapies involve the use of specific herbs, treatments, and practices to rejuvenate the body, enhance immunity, and promote overall well-being. Rasayana herbs such as Ashwagandha, Shatavari, and Guduchi are particularly beneficial for supporting men's health and vitality.

Preventive Measures and Maintenance

In Ayurveda, prevention is considered the best approach to maintaining health and preventing disease. By adopting preventive measures and regular maintenance practices, men can support their health and vitality throughout life.

- **Balanced Diet:** A balanced and nourishing diet is essential for maintaining health and preventing disease. Ayurveda recommends a diet that is appropriate for your dosha constitution and season, focusing on fresh, organic, and whole foods. Avoiding processed foods, refined sugars, and unhealthy fats is also important for preventing disease and maintaining vitality.

- **Regular Exercise:** Regular physical activity is essential for maintaining health and preventing disease. Ayurveda recommends that men engage in exercises that are appropriate for their dosha constitution and fitness goals. Regular exercise helps to boost energy levels, support muscle mass, and maintain cardiovascular health.

- **Detoxification:** Regular detoxification is important for maintaining health and preventing the buildup of toxins (Ama) in the body. Ayurveda recommends seasonal detox practices such as Panchakarma, as well as daily detox practices such as oil pulling, dry brushing, and the use of detoxifying herbs such as Triphala.

- **Sleep and Rest:** Adequate sleep and rest are essential for maintaining health and preventing disease. Ayurveda emphasizes the importance of a regular sleep schedule and creating a calming bedtime routine to promote restful sleep. Herbs such as Ashwagandha and Jatamansi can also support sleep and relaxation.

By adopting these preventive measures and maintenance practices, men can support their health, prevent disease, and enjoy a long, healthy, and fulfilling life.

In this chapter, we have explored the unique health needs of men in Ayurveda, focusing on energy, vitality, reproductive health, and hormonal balance. We also discussed Ayurvedic strategies for men, including diet, exercise, herbal support, and treatments. Finally, we provided guidance on promoting longevity and lifelong health through preventive measures and regular maintenance practices.

As we move forward, our focus will shift to the younger generation, exploring how the wisdom of Ayurveda can be applied to nurture the health and development of children. By understanding the principles that support their physical, mental, and emotional growth, you can lay a strong foundation for their future well-being, helping them to thrive in a balanced and holistic way from an early age.

Chapter 12: Ayurveda for Children

Children's health in Ayurveda is viewed with great care and consideration, focusing on nurturing growth, development, and well-being from infancy through adolescence. Ayurveda emphasizes the importance of a balanced lifestyle, proper nutrition, and a supportive environment to ensure that children thrive physically, mentally, and emotionally. This chapter will explore Ayurvedic principles for children's health, offer guidance on creating a healthy environment through diet, routine, and structure, and provide safe and effective herbal remedies and treatments that can be integrated into parenting. By adopting these Ayurvedic practices, parents can support their children's holistic development and lay the foundation for a healthy and balanced life.

Ayurvedic Principles for Children's Health

Growth and Development

In Ayurveda, children's health is closely linked to the concept of "Swastha," which means a state of balance and well-being. The early years of life are seen as a critical period for establishing a strong foundation for future health. During this time, the focus is on supporting the natural growth and development of the child's body and mind while ensuring that the doshas remain balanced.

- **Kapha Stage of Life:** Ayurveda teaches that the early years of childhood, from birth to around age 16, are predominantly governed by Kapha dosha. Kapha is associated with growth, strength, and stability, which are essential for the physical and mental development of children. This stage of life is characterized by rapid growth, the building of tissues, and the development of the immune system. To support this growth, children need nourishing foods, adequate sleep, and a stable routine that fosters both physical and emotional security.

- **Balancing the Doshas:** While Kapha is the dominant dosha during childhood, it is important to maintain balance among all three doshas—Vata, Pitta, and Kapha—to ensure healthy growth and development. For example, an excess of Kapha can lead to conditions such as weight gain, respiratory issues, and lethargy, while an imbalance in Vata may result in anxiety, restlessness, and irregular sleep patterns. Pitta imbalances can cause irritability, skin rashes, and digestive issues. Ayurvedic practices help to keep the doshas balanced by tailoring diet, lifestyle, and environment to the child's individual constitution.

Common Childhood Ailments

Children are prone to various common ailments as their bodies and immune systems develop. Ayurveda provides natural and gentle remedies to address these issues while supporting the body's natural healing processes.

- **Digestive Issues:** Digestive health is crucial for overall well-being in children. Common digestive issues in childhood include colic, constipation, diarrhea, and indigestion. Ayurveda emphasizes the importance of a balanced diet, appropriate portion sizes, and regular meal times to support digestion. Herbal teas made from fennel, ginger, or cumin can help to soothe digestive discomfort, while ghee and warm milk can be used to ease constipation.

- **Respiratory Infections:** Respiratory issues such as colds, coughs, and congestion are common in children, particularly during the Kapha stage of life. Ayurveda recommends the use of warm, spicy foods, such as ginger and turmeric, to help clear congestion and support the respiratory system. Nasya (nasal administration of herbal oils) can also be used to keep the nasal passages clear and support respiratory health.

- **Skin Conditions:** Skin conditions such as rashes, eczema, and dry skin are common in children and are often related to imbalances in Pitta and Vata doshas. Ayurvedic treatments for skin conditions include the use of cooling and soothing herbs such as neem and aloe vera, as well as regular oil massage (Abhyanga) with coconut or almond oil to keep the skin hydrated and healthy.

- **Sleep Disturbances:** Sleep is essential for the growth and development of children, and sleep disturbances can have a significant impact on their health. Ayurveda recommends establishing a consistent bedtime routine, including practices such as warm baths, gentle oil massage, and the use of calming herbs like Brahmi or Jatamansi to promote restful sleep.

By understanding these common childhood ailments and applying Ayurvedic remedies, parents can support their children's health naturally and effectively.

Creating a Healthy Environment

Diet and Nutrition for Children

Nutrition plays a vital role in children's health and development. Ayurveda emphasizes the importance of providing children with a balanced and nourishing diet that supports their growth, strengthens their immune system, and keeps their doshas in balance.

- **Nourishing Foods:** Ayurveda recommends a diet rich in fresh, organic, and seasonal foods for children. Whole grains, vegetables, fruits, legumes, nuts, and seeds provide essential nutrients for growth and development. Dairy products such as milk, ghee, and yogurt are also important for supporting bone health and overall vitality. It is important to ensure that meals are well-cooked and easy to digest, avoiding overly spicy, salty, or processed foods that can disrupt digestion and lead to imbalances.

- **Portion Control and Meal Timing:** Proper portion sizes and regular meal times are essential for maintaining balance in children. Ayurveda suggests that children should eat meals at regular intervals, with breakfast being the largest meal of the day to provide energy for growth and activity. Avoiding excessive snacking and ensuring that meals are balanced and nutritious can help prevent digestive issues and support healthy growth.

- **Hydration:** Adequate hydration is essential for children's health, as it supports digestion, circulation, and overall well-being. Ayurveda recommends that children drink warm water or herbal teas throughout the day to stay hydrated. Avoiding sugary drinks and excessive consumption of cold beverages can help maintain balance and support digestion.

Building Routine and Structure

Establishing a consistent routine is crucial for children's physical and emotional development. A structured routine provides children with a sense of security and helps to regulate their energy levels, mood, and overall health.

- **Daily Routine (Dinacharya):** A daily routine, or Dinacharya, is essential for maintaining balance and well-being in children. This routine should include regular meal times, physical activity, and self-care practices. For example, starting the day with a warm bath, followed by a nutritious breakfast and some physical activity, can help set a positive tone for the day. Bedtime routines, such as reading a book, gentle massage, and calming herbal teas, can promote restful sleep and emotional security.

- **Physical Activity:** Regular physical activity is important for children's growth, development, and overall well-being. Ayurveda recommends that children engage in activities that are appropriate for their age and dosha constitution. For example, Vata children may benefit from grounding activities such as yoga or walking, while Pitta children may enjoy swimming or playing sports. Kapha children may need more stimulating activities, such as running or dancing, to maintain energy levels and prevent lethargy.

- **Emotional Support:** Emotional support is essential for children's mental and emotional health. Ayurveda emphasizes the importance of creating a nurturing and supportive environment that allows children to express their emotions and feel secure. Practices such as mindfulness, meditation, and spending time in nature can help children develop emotional resilience and a sense of inner peace.

By creating a healthy environment that includes a balanced diet, regular routine, and emotional support, parents can help their children thrive physically, mentally, and emotionally.

Herbal Remedies and Treatments

Safe and Effective Options

Ayurveda offers a variety of safe and effective herbal remedies and treatments for children. These remedies are designed to support the body's natural healing processes and address common childhood ailments without causing side effects.

- **Herbal Teas:** Herbal teas are a gentle and effective way to support children's health. For example, fennel tea can be used to soothe digestive discomfort, while chamomile tea is calming and promotes restful sleep. Ginger tea can help to relieve cold symptoms and support respiratory health. It is important to use age-appropriate dosages and consult with an Ayurvedic practitioner before introducing new herbs to children.

- **Chyawanprash:** Chyawanprash is a traditional Ayurvedic herbal jam that is particularly beneficial for children's health. It is rich in antioxidants, vitamins, and minerals, and supports immunity, digestion, and overall vitality. Chyawanprash can be given to children daily as a supplement to support growth and development.

- **Ghee:** Ghee is a nourishing and versatile remedy that can be used to support children's health in various ways. It can be added to food to enhance digestion, used as a base for herbal remedies, or applied topically to soothe dry skin or rashes. Ghee is particularly beneficial for balancing Vata dosha and supporting overall health and vitality.

- **Abhyanga (Self-Massage):** Regular oil massage (Abhyanga) is highly recommended for children's health. Abhyanga helps to nourish the skin, improve circulation, and promote relaxation. It is particularly beneficial for balancing Vata dosha and supporting physical and emotional well-being. Coconut oil, almond oil, or sesame oil can be used for massage, depending on the child's dosha constitution.

Integrating Ayurveda into Parenting

Integrating Ayurveda into parenting involves applying Ayurvedic principles to daily life in a way that supports the health and well-being of both the child and the parent. This holistic approach emphasizes the importance of balance, nurturing, and mindful living.

- **Mindful Parenting:** Mindful parenting involves being present and attentive to the needs of your child while also taking care of your own well-being. Ayurveda encourages parents to practice mindfulness, meditation, and self-care to maintain balance and reduce stress. By modeling these practices, parents can create a positive and nurturing environment for their children.

- **Ayurvedic Education:** Teaching children about Ayurveda and the importance of balance, nutrition, and self-care can empower them to make healthy choices as they grow. Simple practices, such as encouraging children to listen to their bodies, choose nourishing foods, and establish a regular routine, can help them develop a strong foundation for lifelong health.

- **Family Rituals:** Incorporating Ayurvedic practices into family rituals can help to create a sense of connection and well-being for everyone. For example, practicing daily Abhyanga together, sharing a healthy meal, or spending time in nature as a family can strengthen bonds and promote overall health and happiness.

By integrating Ayurveda into parenting, parents can support their children's holistic development and create a nurturing environment that fosters physical, mental, and emotional well-being.

In this chapter, we have explored Ayurvedic principles for children's health, focusing on growth and development, common childhood ailments, and creating a healthy environment through diet, routine, and structure. We also discussed safe and effective herbal remedies and treatments, as well as strategies for integrating Ayurveda into parenting. By adopting these Ayurvedic practices, parents can support their children's holistic development and lay the foundation for a healthy and balanced life.

As we move forward, we will shift our focus to the wisdom Ayurveda offers for embracing the later stages of life. Aging gracefully is a journey that involves maintaining vitality, balance, and a deep sense of well-being. Through Ayurvedic practices, you can learn to navigate the natural process of aging with strength, wisdom, and grace, continuing to live a vibrant and fulfilling life at every stage.

Chapter 13:
Aging Gracefully with Ayurveda

Aging is a natural and inevitable part of life, and Ayurveda offers a holistic approach to embracing this process with grace and vitality. Rather than viewing aging as a decline, Ayurveda sees it as a stage of life where wisdom, experience, and spiritual growth come to the forefront. The key to aging gracefully lies in maintaining balance and vitality throughout life, using diet, lifestyle practices, and herbal support to address the changes that come with age. In this chapter, we will explore the Ayurvedic perspective on aging, discuss practices for healthy aging, and provide guidance on addressing common age-related issues such as joint health and cognitive function. By integrating these Ayurvedic principles, you can navigate the aging process with confidence and well-being.

Ayurvedic Perspective on Aging

Embracing the Aging Process

In Ayurveda, the process of aging is viewed through the lens of the doshas and the concept of "Vata Kala," the stage of life dominated by Vata dosha. As we age, Vata's qualities of dryness, lightness, and mobility become more prominent, which can lead to certain physical and mental challenges if not properly balanced. However, Ayurveda also recognizes that aging is a time of increased wisdom, spiritual growth, and the opportunity to cultivate inner peace.

- **Vata and Aging:** As Vata dosha becomes more dominant with age, it can lead to increased dryness in the skin and tissues, joint stiffness, and a general decrease in physical strength and stamina. Mentally, an increase in Vata can manifest as restlessness, anxiety, and forgetfulness. However, by balancing Vata through diet, lifestyle, and herbal practices, these challenges can be mitigated, allowing for a more graceful aging process.

- **Wisdom and Spiritual Growth:** Ayurveda views aging as a time to embrace wisdom and spiritual growth. The later years of life are seen as an opportunity to focus on self-reflection, spiritual practices, and the cultivation of inner peace. This stage of life is also a time to share knowledge and experience with younger generations, contributing to the continuity of wisdom and tradition.

Embracing the aging process with a positive and proactive mindset, rather than resisting it, allows for a more fulfilling and enriched experience of life's later stages.

Maintaining Balance and Vitality

Maintaining balance and vitality as we age is essential for enjoying good health and well-being. Ayurveda emphasizes the importance of keeping the doshas in balance, particularly Vata, to prevent the common issues associated with aging.

- **Balancing Vata:** Since Vata dosha becomes more prominent with age, it is crucial to focus on practices that balance Vata and counteract its drying, light, and mobile qualities. This includes consuming warm, nourishing foods, maintaining a regular routine, and engaging in grounding activities such as yoga and meditation.

- **Supporting Ojas:** Ojas, the vital essence that sustains life, is considered the foundation of physical and mental health in Ayurveda. As we age, it is important to nurture and protect Ojas to maintain vitality, immunity, and overall well-being. This can be achieved through a nourishing diet, regular rest, and the use of rejuvenating herbs and therapies.

- **Promoting Agni:** Agni, the digestive fire, tends to weaken with age, leading to issues such as poor digestion, low energy, and a decrease in metabolism. Maintaining a strong Agni is essential for overall health and vitality. Ayurveda recommends consuming easily digestible foods, avoiding heavy and processed foods, and incorporating digestive spices such as ginger, cumin, and turmeric into the diet.

By focusing on these principles, you can maintain balance and vitality throughout the aging process, allowing for a healthy and fulfilling life.

Practices for Healthy Aging

Diet, Exercise, and Lifestyle

A healthy diet, regular exercise, and a balanced lifestyle are the cornerstones of aging gracefully with Ayurveda. By adopting these practices, you can support your body and mind as you age, promoting longevity and overall well-being.

- **Nourishing Diet:** A balanced and nourishing diet is essential for healthy aging. Ayurveda recommends consuming warm, cooked foods that are easy to digest and rich in nutrients. Focus on whole grains, fresh vegetables, fruits, legumes, nuts, seeds, and dairy products such as milk and ghee. Avoid cold, raw, and processed foods, which can aggravate Vata and weaken digestion. Hydration is also important, so drink plenty of warm water and herbal teas throughout the day.

- **Herbs and Spices:** Certain herbs and spices can support healthy aging by enhancing digestion, boosting immunity, and promoting vitality. Include digestive spices such as ginger, turmeric, cumin, and coriander in your meals. Rejuvenating herbs such as Ashwagandha, Shatavari, and Guduchi can help to maintain strength, energy, and overall health as you age.

- **Regular Exercise:** Regular physical activity is important for maintaining strength, flexibility, and overall vitality as you age. Ayurveda recommends gentle exercises that are appropriate for your dosha constitution and physical capabilities. Yoga, walking, swimming, and tai chi are all excellent options for staying active while minimizing strain on the joints and muscles. Regular exercise also helps to keep the mind sharp and supports emotional well-being.

- **Routine and Rest:** Establishing a consistent daily routine, or Dinacharya, is essential for maintaining balance and well-being as you age. This routine should include regular mealtimes, physical activity, and self-care practices. Adequate rest and sleep are also crucial for healthy aging, as they allow the body and mind to rejuvenate. Ayurveda recommends going to bed early and waking up early to align with the body's natural rhythms.

- **Mental and Emotional Health:** Maintaining mental and emotional health is key to aging gracefully. Engage in activities that stimulate the mind, such as reading, puzzles, or learning new skills. Meditation, mindfulness, and spending time in nature can help to reduce stress, promote emotional balance, and support spiritual growth.

Herbal Support for Longevity

Ayurveda offers a variety of herbs that are specifically recommended for promoting longevity and vitality as you age. These herbs help to nourish the body, support the immune system, and maintain physical and mental health.

- **Ashwagandha:** Ashwagandha is a powerful adaptogen that supports overall vitality, reduces stress, and enhances energy levels. It is particularly beneficial for balancing Vata dosha and promoting strength and endurance. Ashwagandha can be taken as a supplement in the form of a powder, capsule, or tincture.

- **Shatavari:** Shatavari is known for its rejuvenating and nourishing properties. It supports hormonal balance, enhances immunity, and promotes vitality. Shatavari is particularly beneficial for maintaining Ojas and overall well-being as you age. It can be taken as a supplement in the form of a powder, capsule, or herbal tea.

- **Guduchi:** Guduchi is an Ayurvedic herb known for its ability to support the immune system, detoxify the body, and promote longevity. It is particularly beneficial for maintaining a strong Agni and supporting overall health. Guduchi can be taken as a supplement in the form of a powder, capsule, or herbal tea.

- **Triphala:** Triphala is a traditional Ayurvedic formula made from three fruits: Amalaki, Bibhitaki, and Haritaki. It is known for its gentle detoxifying and rejuvenating effects. Triphala supports digestion, promotes regularity, and helps to maintain overall health as you age. It can be taken as a supplement in the form of a powder, capsule, or tea.

- **Brahmi:** Brahmi is an Ayurvedic herb that supports cognitive function, memory, and mental clarity. It is particularly beneficial for maintaining mental sharpness and preventing cognitive decline as you age. Brahmi can be taken as a supplement in the form of a powder, capsule, or herbal tea.

These herbs, when used as part of a holistic Ayurvedic approach, can help to support longevity, vitality, and overall well-being as you age.

Addressing Common Age-Related Issues

Joint Health and Mobility

Joint health and mobility are common concerns as we age, particularly as Vata dosha becomes more dominant. Ayurveda offers specific strategies and remedies to support joint health, reduce stiffness, and maintain mobility.

- **Diet for Joint Health:** A diet that supports joint health is essential for maintaining mobility and reducing inflammation. Ayurveda recommends consuming warm, nourishing foods that are rich in healthy fats, such as ghee, sesame oil, and olive oil. Anti-inflammatory foods such as turmeric, ginger, and leafy greens are also beneficial. Avoid cold, raw, and processed foods that can aggravate Vata and contribute to joint stiffness.

- **Herbal Remedies:** Specific Ayurvedic herbs can help to support joint health and reduce inflammation. Guggulu, an Ayurvedic resin, is known for its anti-inflammatory properties and is particularly beneficial for joint health. Ashwagandha and Shatavari also support joint health by promoting strength and reducing inflammation. These herbs can be taken as supplements or used in herbal formulations.

- **Abhyanga (Self-Massage):** Regular oil massage (Abhyanga) is highly recommended for maintaining joint health and mobility as you age. Using warm sesame oil or a medicated Ayurvedic oil, massage the joints and muscles daily to improve circulation, reduce stiffness, and promote flexibility. Abhyanga is particularly beneficial for balancing Vata dosha and supporting overall mobility.

- **Exercise and Movement:** Regular physical activity is important for maintaining joint health and mobility. Ayurveda recommends gentle exercises such as yoga, walking, and swimming to keep the joints flexible and reduce stiffness. Specific yoga poses, such as Warrior Pose (Virabhadrasana) and Tree Pose (Vrksasana), can help to strengthen the joints and improve balance.

Cognitive Function and Memory

Maintaining cognitive function and memory is essential for healthy aging. Ayurveda offers specific practices and herbs to support mental clarity, enhance memory, and prevent cognitive decline.

- **Diet for Cognitive Health:** A diet that supports cognitive health is essential for maintaining mental clarity and memory as you age. Ayurveda recommends consuming nutrient-dense foods that nourish the brain, such as almonds, walnuts, avocados, and leafy greens. Healthy fats, such as ghee and coconut oil, are also important for supporting cognitive function. Avoid processed foods, excessive sugar, and stimulants, which can impair cognitive function and contribute to mental fog.

- **Herbal Support:** Specific Ayurvedic herbs are known for their ability to support cognitive function and memory. Brahmi is one of the most important herbs for mental clarity and memory. It supports cognitive function, enhances memory, and promotes mental agility. Shankhapushpi is another Ayurvedic herb that supports cognitive function and helps to reduce stress and anxiety. These herbs can be taken as supplements or used in herbal formulations.

- **Mental Stimulation:** Regular mental stimulation is important for maintaining cognitive function and memory as you age. Engage in activities that challenge the mind, such as reading, puzzles, or learning new skills. Ayurveda also recommends practices such as meditation and mindfulness to enhance mental clarity and focus.

- **Rest and Relaxation:** Adequate rest and relaxation are essential for maintaining cognitive function and memory. Ayurveda recommends getting regular sleep, practicing meditation, and engaging in activities that promote relaxation and reduce stress. Herbs such as Ashwagandha and Jatamansi can also support restful sleep and relaxation.

By addressing common age-related issues such as joint health and cognitive function through Ayurvedic practices, you can maintain mobility, mental clarity, and overall well-being as you age.

In this chapter, we have explored the Ayurvedic perspective on aging, focusing on embracing the aging process, maintaining balance and vitality, and promoting healthy aging through diet, exercise, lifestyle, and herbal support. We also discussed strategies for addressing common age-related issues such as joint health and cognitive function. By integrating these Ayurvedic principles and practices, you can navigate the aging process with grace, vitality, and well-being.

As we move forward, we will explore how to integrate Ayurvedic wisdom into the fabric of modern living. This includes adapting ancient practices to fit the demands of today's busy world, creating a harmonious home environment, and balancing technology with mindful living. By doing so, you can bring the timeless principles of Ayurveda into every aspect of your life, ensuring that you remain balanced, centered, and well in the midst of contemporary challenges.

Chapter 14:
Ayurveda in Modern Living

In today's fast-paced world, the ancient wisdom of Ayurveda offers a path to balance, health, and well-being amidst the challenges of modern life. While Ayurveda is rooted in principles that date back thousands of years, its teachings remain profoundly relevant and adaptable to contemporary living. This chapter explores how to apply Ayurvedic principles in a busy world, create a balanced home environment, and integrate technology with Ayurvedic practices. By embracing Ayurveda in modern living, you can achieve greater harmony in your daily life and enhance your overall well-being.

Applying Ayurveda in a Busy World

Adapting Ancient Wisdom to Modern Life

The core principles of Ayurveda—balance, natural rhythms, and holistic health—are timeless, but applying them in the context of a busy, modern lifestyle can seem challenging. However, with some thoughtful adaptation, you can integrate Ayurveda into your daily routine, no matter how hectic your life may be.

- **Morning Routine (Dinacharya):** Establishing a consistent morning routine is a foundational practice in Ayurveda. Even with a busy schedule, dedicating time each morning to self-care can set a positive tone for the day. Start your day with practices such as tongue scraping, oil pulling, and drinking warm water with lemon to cleanse and hydrate the body. Follow with a few minutes of meditation or deep breathing exercises to center the mind. If time allows, incorporate a short yoga practice or gentle stretching to awaken the body.

- **Mindful Eating:** In a world where fast food and eating on the go are common, Ayurveda encourages mindful eating as a way to nourish both body and mind. Even during busy days, try to create space for meals without distractions, such as phones or computers. Focus on the taste, texture, and aroma of your food, and chew slowly to aid digestion. Opt for warm, cooked meals that are easy to digest and aligned with your dosha, and avoid skipping meals or eating late at night.

- **Balancing Work and Rest:** Modern life often involves long hours at work, but maintaining a balance between work and rest is essential for health. Ayurveda emphasizes the importance of regular breaks to avoid burnout and maintain mental clarity. Incorporate short breaks throughout your workday to stretch, walk, or practice deep breathing. Prioritize rest in the evenings by creating a calming bedtime routine, such as drinking herbal tea, practicing Abhyanga (self-massage with warm oil), and disconnecting from digital devices.

- **Adapting Ayurvedic Practices:** While some traditional Ayurvedic practices may seem time-consuming, they can be adapted to fit into a modern lifestyle. For example, if you cannot perform a full Abhyanga every day, consider doing a quick self-massage of the hands, feet, and scalp before bed. If you don't have time for a full yoga session, try a few key poses that balance your dosha. The key is to incorporate these practices in a way that is sustainable and supportive of your lifestyle.

By adapting ancient Ayurvedic wisdom to the demands of modern life, you can create a sense of balance and well-being that supports your overall health.

Overcoming Common Challenges

Integrating Ayurveda into modern living can present certain challenges, particularly when it comes to maintaining consistency and adapting practices to a busy schedule. However, with some practical strategies, these challenges can be overcome.

- **Time Management:** One of the most common challenges is finding the time to incorporate Ayurvedic practices into your daily routine. To address this, prioritize the most important practices and start with small, manageable steps. For example, begin with a simple morning routine, such as drinking warm water with lemon and practicing five minutes of meditation. Gradually add more practices as you become comfortable. Use a planner or digital tools to schedule time for self-care, just as you would for other important tasks.

- **Consistency:** Maintaining consistency can be difficult, especially when life gets busy. To stay consistent, make Ayurvedic practices part of your daily routine by associating them with existing habits. For example, practice deep breathing while waiting for your morning coffee to brew or perform a quick self-massage before brushing your teeth at night. Consistency is key to reaping the full benefits of Ayurveda, so aim to incorporate these practices into your life in a sustainable way.

- **Social and Environmental Factors:** Social and environmental factors, such as eating out, social events, or work commitments, can make it challenging to follow Ayurvedic guidelines. When dining out, choose meals that align with your dosha and avoid heavy, processed, or overly spicy foods. If social events disrupt your routine, return to your Ayurvedic practices the next day. Create a supportive environment at home by stocking your kitchen with Ayurvedic staples, such as spices, herbs, and ghee, and setting up a dedicated space for yoga and meditation.

- **Mindset and Flexibility:** Adopting Ayurveda requires a mindset of flexibility and self-compassion. It's important to remember that Ayurveda is not about perfection but about creating balance in a way that works for you. Be patient with yourself as you integrate these practices, and allow for flexibility as life circumstances change. The goal is to cultivate a sense of well-being and harmony, even in the midst of a busy life.

By addressing these common challenges, you can successfully integrate Ayurveda into your modern lifestyle and enjoy its many benefits.

Creating a Balanced Home Environment

Ayurvedic Principles for Home Design

Your home environment plays a significant role in your overall well-being. In Ayurveda, the principles of "Vastu Shastra," a traditional system of architecture, offer guidance on creating harmonious living spaces that promote health, balance, and positive energy. While Vastu is a comprehensive and detailed practice, you can incorporate its basic principles to create a balanced and supportive home environment.

- **Natural Light and Airflow:** Ensure that your home is well-ventilated and receives plenty of natural light. Fresh air and sunlight are essential for maintaining a healthy environment and promoting positive energy. Open windows regularly to allow fresh air to circulate, and use light, airy curtains to maximize natural light. Consider placing plants around your home to improve air quality and bring in natural elements.

- **Space and Clutter:** A cluttered space can create mental and physical stagnation, while a clean, organized environment promotes clarity and peace. Ayurveda recommends decluttering your living spaces to remove excess items and create a sense of openness and flow. Use natural materials, such as wood, stone, and cotton, to create a grounding and calming atmosphere.

- **Colors and Elements:** The colors and elements used in your home can influence your mood and energy levels. Ayurveda suggests using colors that align with your dosha and promote balance. For example, Vata types may benefit from warm, grounding colors like earthy tones, while Pitta types may find cooling colors like blue and green more calming. Kapha types may prefer invigorating colors like warm yellows and oranges. Incorporate the five elements—earth, water, fire, air, and space—into your home design to create a balanced environment.

- **Room Functionality:** Each room in your home should be designed with its specific function in mind. For example, the kitchen, where food is prepared, should be clean, well-organized, and filled with nourishing ingredients. The bedroom, a space for rest and rejuvenation, should be free from distractions, such as electronic devices, and decorated with calming colors and soft textures. The living room, a space for socializing and relaxation, should be inviting and comfortable, with plenty of seating and warm lighting.

Mindful Living Spaces

Creating mindful living spaces involves designing your home environment to support relaxation, focus, and overall well-being. This includes creating areas for meditation, yoga, and other self-care practices, as well as fostering a sense of peace and harmony throughout your home.

- **Meditation Space:** Designate a quiet and peaceful area in your home for meditation and mindfulness practices. This space should be free from distractions and clutter, with comfortable seating, soft lighting, and calming colors. You might include elements like cushions, candles, and incense to create a soothing atmosphere. Make this space a sanctuary where you can retreat for daily meditation and reflection.

- **Yoga Space:** If possible, set aside a dedicated space for yoga practice. This area should be spacious enough for your yoga mat and allow for free movement. Use natural materials, such as a cotton or jute yoga mat, and incorporate elements like plants, crystals, or artwork that inspire you. Keep the space clean and uncluttered, and ensure that it is well-ventilated and filled with natural light.

- **Calming Corners:** Create small calming corners throughout your home where you can relax and unwind. These spaces might include a comfortable chair with a cozy blanket, a reading nook with soft lighting, or a window seat with a view of nature. Use these spaces to take a break from the busyness of daily life, read a book, or simply sit and breathe.

- **Sacred Objects:** Incorporate sacred objects, such as statues, crystals, or meaningful artwork, into your living spaces to create a sense of spirituality and connection. These objects can serve as reminders of your intentions and help you stay grounded and centered throughout the day.

By creating mindful living spaces, you can cultivate a home environment that supports your well-being and enhances your daily Ayurvedic practices.

Technology and Ayurveda

Balancing Digital Detox with Ayurvedic Practices

In the modern world, technology plays an integral role in daily life, but excessive use of digital devices can lead to imbalances, particularly in Vata dosha. Ayurveda emphasizes the importance of balancing technology use with digital detox practices to maintain mental clarity, reduce stress, and promote overall well-being.

- **Digital Detox:** A digital detox involves taking intentional breaks from digital devices, such as smartphones, computers, and televisions, to reduce mental and sensory overload. Ayurveda recommends incorporating regular digital detox periods into your routine, such as disconnecting from devices during meals, setting boundaries around screen time in the evening, and taking technology-free weekends or vacations. Use these times to engage in mindful activities, such as reading, meditation, spending time in nature, or connecting with loved ones.

- **Mindful Technology Use:** When using technology, practice mindfulness to reduce the negative impact on your well-being. This includes being aware of your posture, taking breaks to stretch and move, and using devices with intention rather than habit. Set boundaries around technology use, such as designating device-free zones in your home or setting specific times for checking email and social media. Use blue light filters on screens in the evening to reduce the impact on sleep, and avoid using devices for at least an hour before bedtime.

- **Grounding Practices:** To counteract the overstimulation caused by excessive technology use, incorporate grounding Ayurvedic practices into your daily routine. These might include self-massage with warm oil (Abhyanga), practicing yoga or tai chi, and spending time outdoors in nature. Grounding practices help to calm the nervous system, reduce Vata imbalances, and promote a sense of peace and stability.

Tools and Apps for Ayurvedic Living

While Ayurveda encourages mindfulness and balance, technology can also be a valuable tool for supporting Ayurvedic living in the modern world. There are a variety of apps and digital tools designed to help you integrate Ayurveda into your daily life, track your progress, and deepen your understanding of Ayurvedic principles.

- **Dosha Quizzes:** Many apps offer dosha quizzes that can help you determine your Ayurvedic constitution and identify any imbalances. Understanding your dosha is the first step to personalizing your Ayurvedic practices, and these quizzes can provide insights into your unique needs.

- **Meditation and Mindfulness Apps:** Apps like Headspace, Calm, and Insight Timer offer guided meditations, mindfulness practices, and breathing exercises that align with Ayurvedic principles. These apps can help you establish a regular meditation practice, reduce stress, and enhance mental clarity.

- **Yoga Apps:** Yoga apps such as YogaGlo, Down Dog, and Asana Rebel offer a wide range of yoga classes that can be tailored to your dosha and fitness level. These apps provide guidance on poses, breathwork, and relaxation techniques, making it easier to incorporate yoga into your daily routine.

- **Ayurvedic Lifestyle Apps:** Apps like Ayurveda Pro, Banyan Botanicals, and Ayurvedic Daily offer personalized Ayurvedic lifestyle recommendations, including diet, exercise, and self-care practices based on your dosha. These apps provide tips on seasonal adjustments, herbal remedies, and routines to support your well-being.

- **Recipe and Nutrition Apps:** Apps such as My Ayurvedic Cookbook and Eat Taste Heal offer Ayurvedic recipes and meal plans that are tailored to your dosha. These apps provide guidance on selecting foods that promote balance and vitality, as well as tips for mindful eating.

By using these tools and apps, you can enhance your Ayurvedic practices, stay motivated, and deepen your understanding of Ayurveda in the context of modern living.

In this chapter, we have explored how to apply Ayurvedic principles in a busy world, focusing on adapting ancient wisdom to modern life and overcoming common challenges. We also discussed creating a balanced home environment through Ayurvedic design principles and mindful living spaces. Additionally, we examined the role of technology in modern living and how to balance digital detox with Ayurvedic practices, as well as tools and apps that can support your Ayurvedic journey.

As we move forward, we will delve deeper into how to fully embrace Ayurvedic wisdom in your everyday life. This final reflection will guide you in making Ayurveda not just a practice, but a way of life—one that continues to grow and evolve with you. By integrating these teachings with intention and commitment, you can create a life of lasting balance, profound health, and true fulfillment, all while remaining connected to the timeless wisdom of Ayurveda.

Chapter 15:
Embracing Ayurvedic Wisdom

Embracing Ayurvedic wisdom is not just about adopting a set of practices; it's about integrating a holistic approach to life that honors the mind, body, and spirit. As you have journeyed through the principles and practices of Ayurveda, the final step is to make Ayurveda a sustainable and enriching part of your daily life. This chapter will guide you on how to personalize your Ayurvedic journey, set meaningful goals, and continue your education and growth in Ayurveda. We will also explore the future of Ayurveda, including innovations, trends, and its global impact. By embracing Ayurvedic wisdom, you can cultivate a life of balance, health, and fulfillment.

Integrating Ayurveda into Your Life

Personalizing Your Ayurvedic Journey

Ayurveda is not a one-size-fits-all system; it is deeply personal and adaptable to your unique constitution, lifestyle, and goals. Integrating Ayurveda into your life involves understanding your dosha, recognizing your current imbalances, and tailoring Ayurvedic practices to meet your specific needs. This personalized approach ensures that Ayurveda becomes a sustainable and enriching part of your daily routine.

- **Understanding Your Dosha:** The first step in personalizing your Ayurvedic journey is to understand your unique dosha constitution (Prakriti) and any current imbalances (Vikriti). By knowing whether you are predominantly Vata, Pitta, Kapha, or a combination of these doshas, you can tailor your diet, lifestyle, and self-care practices to support balance and well-being. For example, if you are primarily Vata, you might focus on grounding practices, warm foods, and a stable routine. If you are Pitta, you may prioritize cooling foods, calming activities, and stress management.

- **Tailoring Your Practices:** Once you understand your dosha, you can begin to tailor Ayurvedic practices to your specific needs. This includes choosing the right foods, exercises, and self-care rituals that align with your constitution. For example, you might choose to incorporate Abhyanga (self-massage) with oils that balance your dosha, practice yoga poses that support your constitution, and select herbs that enhance your overall vitality. Personalizing these practices ensures that Ayurveda fits seamlessly into your life.

- **Adapting to Life Stages and Seasons:** Ayurveda teaches that your dosha balance can change throughout life's stages and seasons. For instance, Vata naturally increases as you age, while Pitta may dominate during mid-life. Similarly, the seasons influence your dosha balance, with Kapha rising in spring, Pitta in summer, and Vata in winter. Adapting your Ayurvedic practices to these changes helps maintain balance and harmony throughout the year and as you move through different phases of life.

Setting Goals and Intentions

Setting goals and intentions is a powerful way to guide your Ayurvedic journey and ensure that you are moving towards greater health, balance, and fulfillment. Goals provide direction, while intentions help you stay aligned with your deeper values and aspirations.

- **Setting Ayurvedic Goals:** Begin by identifying specific health and wellness goals that align with your Ayurvedic journey. These might include improving digestion, reducing stress, increasing energy levels, or achieving better sleep. Be specific about what you want to achieve and set realistic, measurable goals. For example, you might set a goal to practice meditation for 10 minutes every morning or to follow a dosha-specific diet for 30 days.

- **Creating a Vision Board:** A vision board is a visual representation of your goals and intentions. It can be a powerful tool to keep you motivated and focused on your Ayurvedic journey. Include images, quotes, and affirmations that inspire you and reflect the life you want to create with Ayurveda. Place your vision board in a space where you will see it daily, such as your meditation area or bedroom.

- **Practicing Intention Setting:** In Ayurveda, setting intentions is about aligning your actions with your higher purpose and values. Each morning, take a few moments to set an intention for the day. This could be as simple as "Today, I will nourish my body with wholesome foods" or "I will approach my work with calm and focus." Setting intentions helps to bring mindfulness to your actions and keeps you aligned with your Ayurvedic goals.

- **Tracking Progress:** Regularly track your progress towards your Ayurvedic goals. Keep a journal where you record your experiences, challenges, and successes. Reflect on how your Ayurvedic practices are impacting your health and well-being, and make adjustments as needed. Celebrate your achievements, no matter how small, and stay committed to your journey.

By setting clear goals and intentions, you can create a roadmap for your Ayurvedic journey that leads to greater health, balance, and fulfillment.

Continuing Education and Growth

Resources for Further Learning

Ayurveda is a vast and rich field of knowledge that offers endless opportunities for learning and growth. Whether you are new to Ayurveda or have been practicing for some time, continuing your education can deepen your understanding and enhance your practice.

- **Books and Literature:** There are numerous books on Ayurveda that cover a wide range of topics, from foundational principles to specific areas like diet, herbs, and yoga. Some recommended books include "The Complete Book of Ayurvedic Home Remedies" by Vasant Lad, "Ayurveda: The Science of Self-Healing" by Dr. Vasant Lad, and "Prakriti: Your Ayurvedic Constitution" by Dr. Robert Svoboda. These books provide valuable insights and practical guidance for incorporating Ayurveda into your life.

- **Online Courses and Workshops:** Many online platforms offer courses and workshops on Ayurveda, ranging from beginner to advanced levels. These courses cover topics such as Ayurvedic nutrition, herbal medicine, yoga, and self-care practices. Look for courses offered by reputable Ayurvedic practitioners and institutions, such as the Ayurvedic Institute, Kripalu, and Banyan Botanicals.

- **Podcasts and Videos:** Podcasts and videos are great resources for learning on the go. There are many Ayurvedic podcasts and YouTube channels that offer valuable information, tips, and interviews with experts in the field. Some popular podcasts include "The

Everyday Ayurveda and Yoga Podcast" and "Ayurveda Life School Podcast." You can also find instructional videos on yoga, meditation, and Ayurvedic cooking.

- **Professional Certification:** If you are passionate about Ayurveda and want to deepen your knowledge, consider pursuing professional certification as an Ayurvedic Health Counselor, Practitioner, or Doctor. Many accredited schools and institutions offer certification programs that provide in-depth training in Ayurvedic principles, diagnostics, and therapies. This path can open up opportunities to share Ayurvedic wisdom with others and contribute to the growing field of holistic health.

Finding Community and Support

Connecting with others who share your interest in Ayurveda can provide support, inspiration, and a sense of community. Whether you are seeking guidance, friendship, or simply a space to share your experiences, finding a community can enrich your Ayurvedic journey.

- **Joining Local Groups:** Many cities have local Ayurvedic groups or meetups where people come together to discuss Ayurveda, practice yoga, and share meals. Joining these groups can provide a sense of belonging and offer opportunities to learn from others. Look for groups on social media platforms like Facebook or Meetup, or check with local yoga studios and wellness centers.

- **Online Communities:** Online communities are a great way to connect with like-minded individuals from around the world. There are numerous online forums,

Facebook groups, and Instagram communities dedicated to Ayurveda. These platforms allow you to ask questions, share your experiences, and receive support from others who are on a similar journey.

- **Attending Retreats and Workshops:** Ayurvedic retreats and workshops offer immersive experiences where you can deepen your practice, learn from experts, and connect with others. Many retreats focus on specific areas of Ayurveda, such as detoxification (Panchakarma), yoga, or meditation. Attending these events can provide a space for personal growth, healing, and rejuvenation.

- **Mentorship:** If you are looking for more personalized guidance, consider finding a mentor or Ayurvedic practitioner who can support you on your journey. A mentor can provide advice, answer questions, and help you navigate challenges as you integrate Ayurveda into your life.

By finding community and support, you can enhance your Ayurvedic journey and build meaningful connections with others who share your passion for holistic health.

The Future of Ayurveda

Innovations and Trends

As Ayurveda continues to grow in popularity around the world, it is evolving in exciting ways. Innovations and trends are emerging that integrate Ayurvedic principles with modern science, technology, and global wellness practices. Understanding these trends can help you stay informed and inspired as you continue your Ayurvedic journey.

- **Ayurvedic Research:** Scientific research on Ayurveda is expanding, with studies exploring the efficacy of Ayurvedic herbs, treatments, and practices in managing various health conditions. This research is helping to bridge the gap between traditional knowledge and modern science, providing evidence-based support for Ayurvedic practices. As more studies are conducted, Ayurveda's credibility in the global health community continues to grow.

- **Personalized Ayurveda:** The concept of personalized medicine is gaining traction, and Ayurveda's focus on individualized treatment is perfectly aligned with this trend. Advances in genetic testing, for example, are allowing practitioners to tailor Ayurvedic recommendations based on an individual's genetic makeup, dosha constitution, and lifestyle. This personalized approach is enhancing the effectiveness of Ayurvedic treatments and making them more accessible to a broader audience.

- **Ayurvedic Skincare and Beauty:** The global beauty industry is increasingly embracing Ayurvedic principles, with a growing demand for natural, herbal-based skincare products. Ayurvedic beauty brands are creating products that harness the power of herbs like turmeric, neem, and sandalwood to promote healthy, radiant skin. This trend reflects a broader movement towards clean, sustainable beauty that aligns with Ayurvedic values.

- **Integration with Modern Wellness Practices:** Ayurveda is being integrated with modern wellness practices, such as functional medicine, yoga therapy, and mindfulness-based stress reduction. This integration is creating a more holistic approach to health and wellness that combines the best of both worlds. As more practitioners and wellness centers adopt Ayurvedic principles, the influence of Ayurveda in the global health landscape continues to expand.

The Global Impact of Ayurvedic Practices

Ayurveda's impact is being felt around the world as more people embrace its holistic approach to health and well-being. This global expansion is fostering cross-cultural exchange, promoting sustainable living, and contributing to the growing movement towards natural and integrative health practices.

- **Cultural Exchange:** As Ayurveda spreads globally, it is fostering cross-cultural exchange and dialogue. Practitioners and enthusiasts from different cultures are sharing their interpretations of Ayurvedic practices, leading to a richer and more diverse understanding of Ayurveda. This exchange is also inspiring new approaches to health and wellness that blend Ayurvedic principles with local traditions and practices.

- **Sustainability and Environmental Awareness:** Ayurveda's emphasis on living in harmony with nature is resonating with the global movement towards sustainability and environmental awareness. Ayurvedic practices, such as using natural remedies, eating seasonally, and reducing waste, are being embraced by those who are committed to sustainable living. This alignment with environmental values is helping to position Ayurveda as a leader in the global wellness movement.

- **Global Health and Wellness:** Ayurveda is contributing to the global health and wellness movement by offering natural, holistic solutions to modern health challenges. Its focus on prevention, personalized care, and mind-body integration is attracting individuals and healthcare practitioners seeking alternatives to conventional medicine. As more people experience the benefits of Ayurveda, its influence on global health continues to grow.

By staying informed about innovations, trends, and the global impact of Ayurveda, you can continue to evolve your practice and contribute to the broader movement towards holistic health.

In this final chapter, we have explored how to integrate Ayurveda into your life by personalizing your journey, setting goals, and continuing your education and growth. We also discussed the future of Ayurveda, including innovations, trends, and its global impact. As you embrace Ayurvedic wisdom, you are not only enhancing your own well-being but also contributing to a global movement that values balance, harmony, and holistic health.

As you move forward on your Ayurvedic journey, remember that Ayurveda is a lifelong path of learning, growth, and self-discovery. By staying connected to your goals, intentions, and community, you can continue to evolve and thrive, embodying the timeless wisdom of Ayurveda in your daily life.

Final Thoughts

As you reach the end of this book, I hope you feel more connected to the wisdom of Ayurveda and how its timeless practices can bring balance, health, and harmony into your everyday life. Ayurveda is not just a set of guidelines—it's a lifestyle that honors the intricate relationship between your body, mind, and spirit. By incorporating these teachings, you've taken the first steps toward living a more vibrant and balanced life.

But remember, this is just the beginning. Ayurveda is a lifelong journey, one of continual learning, growth, and discovery. The practices you've explored in these pages are meant to evolve with you. Whether you're fine-tuning your diet, enhancing your daily routines, or embracing herbal remedies, each small step you take is a powerful move toward deeper well-being.

Want More Holistic Insights?
Sign Up and Get Your Free Ebook!

Let's keep this journey going! By signing up for my mailing list, you'll receive exclusive tips, updates on future books, and practical guidance to support your wellness journey. Plus, as a thank you, you'll get a free ebook—*"Aroma Bliss: 30 Essential Oil Recipes for Home, Body, and Mind."* This collection of simple yet powerful recipes will help you incorporate the healing benefits of essential oils into your life.

Just head over to my website to subscribe and start embracing even more holistic practices!

https://www.serenitysagewood.com

Your Feedback Is Valued!

If *Ayurvedic Wisdom: Balancing Body, Mind, and Spirit* has enriched your life, I'd love to hear your thoughts! Your review not only helps others discover the book but also strengthens our community of like-minded individuals seeking balance and healing. Your words have the power to inspire others to begin their own wellness journey. Please head over to Amazon & Goodreads and let me know what you thought!

Explore More of My Books

If you're looking to further deepen your connection to holistic health, I invite you to explore my other books, each offering unique insights and practical tools to enhance your well-being:

- **Beyond Conventional: The Complete Guide to Alternative and Holistic Health**
  A deeper dive into alternative health practices that go beyond the ordinary, helping you discover new ways to live a balanced, healthy life.

- **Scent to Heal: Comprehensive Guide to Aromatherapy**
  Unlock the healing power of essential oils and learn how to use them to boost physical, emotional, and spiritual health.

These books are designed to provide you with the tools to continue your journey toward balance, vitality, and a deeper connection to yourself.

A Heartfelt Thank You

Thank you from the bottom of my heart for joining me on this journey. Your openness to exploring the wisdom of Ayurveda is truly inspiring. I hope this book has not only empowered you to take control of your health but also offered you peace, clarity, and a deeper connection to your body and spirit.

As you continue to grow and evolve, I encourage you to stay curious, embrace change, and honor your path. Together, we can continue to build a community that supports each other in healing, balance, and holistic well-being.

Wishing you continued health, happiness, and peace,

Serenity Sagewood

Serenity Sagewood

www.ingramcontent.com/pod-product-compliance
Lightning Source LLC
Chambersburg PA
CBHW052204220526
45471CB00004B/1815